TRAEGER GRILL
&
SMOKER COOKBOOK

The Ultimate Guide to Mastering your Pellet Grill with Appetizing Recipes, Plus Tips and Techniques to Earn Pitmaster Status Among your Friends and Families

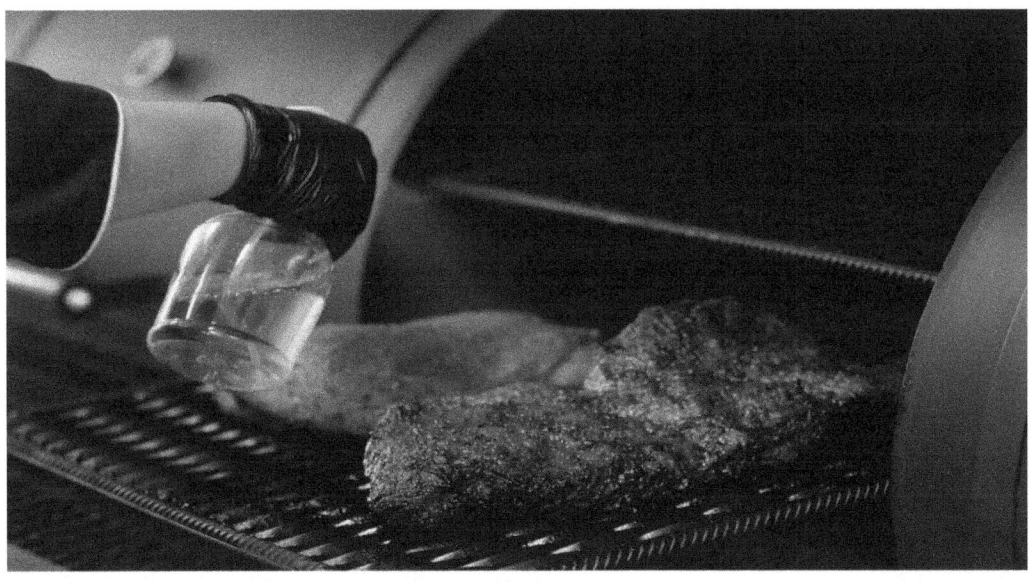

By **MIKE PHELLIS**

© COPYRIGHT 2020, MIKE PHELLIS

ALL RIGHTS RESERVED

This report is towards furnishing precise and dependable data concerning the point and issue secured. The production is available with the possibility that the distributor isn't required to render bookkeeping, formally allowed, or something else, qualified administrations. On the off chance that persuasion is essential, lawful, or proficient; an experienced individual in the area ought to be requested.

The Declaration of Principles, which the American Bar Association Committee and the Publishers and Associations Committee have accepted and supported. Not the slightest bit is it lawful to replicate, copy, or transmit any piece of this report in either electronic methods or the printed group. Recording of this distribution is carefully disallowed, and any capacity of this report isn't permitted except if with composed authorization from the distributor. All rights reserved.

The data given in this is expressed to be honest, and predictable, in that any risk, as far as absentmindedness or something else, by any utilization or maltreatment of any approaches, procedures, or bearings contained inside is the singular and articulate obligation of the beneficiary per user. By no means will any lawful obligation or fault be held against the distributor for any reparation, harms, or money-related misfortune because of the data in this book, either straightforwardly or by implication.

Particular creators claim all copyrights not held by the distributor.

The data in this is offered for educational purposes exclusively and is all-inclusive as so. The introduction of the data is without a contract or any assurance confirmation.

The marks used shall be without consent, and the distribution of the mark shall be without the consent or support of the proprietor of the mark. All trademarks and trademarks within this book are just for explanation and are held clearly by the owners, who are not associated with this record.

TABLE OF CONTENTS

- INTRODUCTION 10
- WOOD PELLETS FOR SMOKING AND GRILLING 11
- WHAT ARE WOOD PELLETS AND HOW ARE THEY MADE? 11
  - FOOD GRADE WOOD PELLETS FOR SMOKING AND GRILLING 12
- WOOD PELLETS AND THE ENVIRONMENT 13
- WOOD PELLET TYPES 15
  - FLAVORED 15
  - BLENDED 16
  - NON-FLAVORED 16
- LOUISIANA GRILLS PELLET FLAVORS GUIDE 17
- THE HISTORY OF PELLET GRILLS & SMOKERS 18
- COMPETITION ARRIVES: THE NEXT GENERATION OF PELLET GRILLS 19
- SET-IT AND FORGET-IT: THE EVOLUTION OF EASE 20
  - BEYOND INDIRECT GRILLING 21
  - THE PLATINUM MARKET 21
  - THE NEW CLASS 21
  - THE FUTURE OF PELLET GRILLS 22
- THE REBIRTH OF TRAEGER 23
- HOW DOES A PELLET SMOKER WORK? 24

- HOW TO USE A PELLET SMOKER TO SMOKE MEAT 24
- ADVANTAGES OF WOOD PELLET SMOKER AND GRILLS 26
- TOP 5 FEATURES SHOULD KNOW BEFORE BUYING PELLET SMOKERS 28
- PELLET SMOKERS BUYING TIPS 30
  - QUALITY CONSTRUCTION 30
  - DURABILITY 30
  - TEMPERATURE RANGE 30
  - PELLET GRILL CONTROLLER 31
  - SIZE AND COOKING AREA 31
- DIFFERENCE BETWEEN PELLET AND THE OTHER GRILLS TYPES EXPLAINED 32
  - CHARCOAL 32
  - GAS 33
  - ELECTRIC 33
  - PELLET 34
  - INFRARED 34
  - CHOOSING THE RIGHT TYPE OF GRILL 35
- WOOD PELLET SMOKER AND GRILL 36
- RECIPES 36
  - 1. TRAEGER BAKED CORN DOG BITES 36
  - 2. BBQ BROWN SUGAR BACON BITES 38
  - 3. SMOKED BEER CHEESE DIP 39
  - 4. ROASTED TINGLE WINGS 41

5. THE DAN PATRICK SHOW GRILLED BLOODY MARY WINGS 42

6. GRILLED SHRIMP TACOS WITH GARLIC CILANTRO LIME SLAW 43

7. BROWN SUGAR AND BACON WRAPPED LIL SMOKIES 45

8. CHINESE JUMBO SHRIMP 46

9. SMOKED ALBACORE TUNA 47

10. TRAEGER SMOKED MUSHROOMS 48

11. TRAEGER SMOKED DEVILED EGGS 49

12. ROASTED TEQUILA-LIME WINGS BY AMANDA HAAS 51

13. BBQ BRISKET HOT DOG 53

14. GRILLED HONEY GARLIC WINGS 54

15. ROASTED ARTICHOKES WITH GARLIC BUTTER 55

16. SMOKED SHRIMP AND GRILLED DUNGENESS CRAB COCKTAIL 56

17. BBQ SPARERIBS WITH SPICY MANDARIN GLAZE 58

18. ROASTED BUFFALO WINGS 59

19. PROSCIUTTO WRAPPED DATES WITH MARCONA ALMONDS..61

20. TEXAS PINTO BEANS BY DOUG SCHEIDING 63

21. STUFFED JALAPENOS 65

22. GRILLED SHRIMP COCKTAIL 66

23. BAKED ARTICHOKE PARMESAN MUSHROOMS 68

24. GRILLED SWEET CAJUN WINGS 69

25. BAKED CAULIFLOWER TOTS 70

26. WILD TURKEY SOUTHWEST EGG ROLLS BY JEREMIAH DOUGHTY 71

27. FOCACCIA 73

28. ROASTED POTATO POUTINE 75

29. SMOKED TROUT DIP 76

30. ROASTED SERRANO WINGS 78

31. WHOLE ROASTED CAULIFLOWER WITH GARLIC PARMESAN BUTTER 80

32. SMOKED BEET-PICKLED EGGS 81

33. BAKED ARTICHOKE DIP 83

34. SMOKED SPICY VENISON JERKY 85

35. GRILLED BISON SLIDERS 87

36. BACON WRAPPED CHICKEN WINGS 88

37. PRETZEL ROLLS 89

38. MINI SAUSAGE ROLLS 91

39. ROASTED SWEET POTATO FRIES 92

40. BRISKET BURNT END NACHOS 93

41. OYSTERS TRAEGEFELLER 95

42. SMOKED TROUT 97

43. TURKEY JALAPEÑO MEATBALLS 98

44. BACON WRAPPED CHERRY TOMATOES 100

45. GRILLED BLOOMING ONION 101

46. EVERYTHING PIGS IN A BLANKET 102

47. SPICY CRAB POPPERS 104

48. THAI CHICKEN SKEWERS 105

49. Prosciutto Wrapped Grilled Shrimp with Peach Salsa 106

50. Smoked Hummus with Roasted Vegetables 107

51. Grilled Korean Short Ribs 109

52. BBQ Chicken Drumsticks 110

53. Smoked Mustard Wings 111

54. Beef Satay 113

55. Baked Sweet Potatoes 114

56. Baked Loaded Tater Tots 115

57. Old Fashioned Cornbread 116

58. Jalapeño Candied Smoked Salmon 117

59. Grilled Corn Salsa 119

60. Traeger Mandarin Wings 120

61. Artichoke & Spinach Dip 121

62. Smoked Dry Rub Wings 123

63. Honey Lime Chicken Adobo Skewers 124

64. Roasted Hasselback Potatoes 125

65. Baked Venison Tater Tot Casserole 127

66. Baked Garlic Parmesan Wings 128

67. Traeger Shrimp 129

68. Grilled Fruit Skewers with Yogurt Sauce 130

69. Grilled Oysters by Journey South 131

70. Double-Decker Pulled Pork Nachos with Smoked Cheese 133

71. Baked Pickles with Buttermilk Dip 134

72. Alder Smoked Scallops with Citrus & Garlic Butter Sauce 136

73. Cold Smoked Cheese 138

74. Tandoori Chicken Wings 139

75. Roasted Jalapeno Cheddar Deviled Eggs 141

76. Garlic Parmesan Chicken Wings 142

The 9 Best Pellet Grills Reviewed 144

1. The Best All-Around Pellet Smoker – Camp Chef SmokePro SG24 Wifi Pellet Grill 144

2. Runner Up – Traeger Pro 575 Wood Pellet Grill 146

3. The Best Budget Pellet Grill – Z Grills ZPG-7002E Wood Pellet Grill & Smoker 147

4. The Best Portable Pellet Smoker – Green Mountain Grills Davy Crockett Wifi Grill 149

5. Best Large Pellet Smoker – Camp Chef SmokePro Lux Pellet Grill 150

6. Camp Chef Woodwind 24 Pellet Grill – A Reliable Mid-Sized Option 151

7. Rec Tec Grills RT-700 Wi-Fi Enabled Wood Pellet Grill – A Tremendous High-End Option 152

8. Pit Boss 700FB Pellet Grill – Large Budget Alternative 153

9. Weber Smokefire – Weber's First Entry into the Pellet Grill Market. 153

Who Pellet Smokers Are Best Suited For? 154

How Pellet Smokers Work 155

Durability and Construction Material 156

- SIZE OF THE HOPPER 156
- PLAN HOW MUCH COOKING REAL ESTATE YOU NEED 157
- COMMON FEATURES AND CAPABILITIES 157
- LENGTH OF WARRANTY 158
- PELLET CONSUMPTION 158
- BEWARE OF GIMMICKS 159
- CUSTOMER SERVICE 159
- PRICE 160
- THE PROS AND CONS OF PURCHASING A SMOKER WITH A PELLET 160
- THERE ARE ALSO A FEW ADVANTAGES UNIQUE TO COOKING WITH A PELLET SMOKER 161

MEAT SMOKING AND GRILLING WITH FLAVORED SMOKE WOODS 162

CONCLUSION 165

INTRODUCTION

*O*ver the last century, barbecues have become outstanding means of getting a social experience and of making healthy delicacies such as chicken and hamburgers grilled on an open grill outside; but, are our current grills our only way to cook our food? While traditional grills are the most famous outdoor cooking systems in our country, they are certainly not the safest or most savory method of grilling our food, which grills are by far the best way to do so.

Wood pellet grills are in several respects preferable to standard grilling with gas and charcoal. The first thing that makes them better over these conventional grills is that you have indirect cooking on pellet grills and so the pellet grills only cook with heated air around your food. No fire emerges from the base of the barbecue or the top of the barbecue, and the cooking is much tastier as smoke and flame cover the meal.

The food cooked in this manner contains a number of carcinogens that are carcinogenic, which occurs because the fat that is existing on the product has already starting to drown when heated, which creates a black crust composed of polycyclic aromatic hydrocarbons which are well-known carcinogenic, however, most people prefer them.

Wood pellet grills have much less carcinogenic items, and most famous companies, including Traeger, make pellet grills with two or more shielding between the food and the heat source, which ensures the possible fat carcinogenic droplets escape out of the chamber into a bucket outside the grill. The extremely harmful fat never gets to the heart center, which is the fuel.

That pellet grills are widely regarded as the best kind of grills to generate smoky foods. If you still wonder how the finest delicacies are made for beef jerky, now you do. Therefore, such forms of grills are very green-friendly as they contain much less greenhouse gas emissions than conventional oil or gas grills. When you cook with them, you have even less of the grill to clean up, because anyone who barbecued knows well that it will take hours to clean the grill after a big barbecue. So, if you decide to purchase a grill and decide to get a backyard pellet barbecue, you'll find a safer option. You're not going to feel sad if you do.

WOOD PELLETS FOR SMOKING AND GRILLING

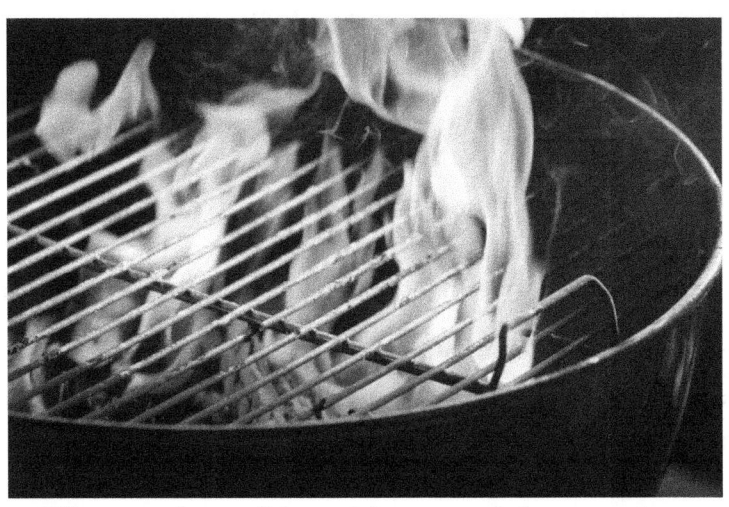

You may have heard a thing or two about pellet grills lately. Maybe your neighbor fired one up while you were over for a football game on Sunday. Or a celebrity you follow on Instagram was describing all the flavor and convenience benefits of smoking meat on a pellet grill.

At Louisiana Grills, we welcome you aboard the Pellet Grill revolution. To understand all things about pellet grilling and smoking, it's essential to understand what fuels these innovative BBQ products. So, we're going to look at wood pellets for smoking and grilling correctly and dive into how they're made, how they stack up against other fuel sources, and which types of wood pellets are the best for smoking and grilling.

WHAT ARE WOOD PELLETS AND HOW ARE THEY MADE?

Wood pellets are the source of fuel for pellets and smokers. Louisiana Grills ® hardwood pellets are produced from 100% raw hardwood, which is processed and ground into sawdust. The dust is then pressurized at high pressure to create small pellets that are powdered and bound together with natural wood lignin. Wood pellets are often regarded as the most available fuel to be found. They contain less than 1% of coal, and the whole 40 lb. bag of pellets can just transform into ½ cup of coal, which will render the air clear. They also have an incredible taste without having to worry about babysitting air to fuel ratios like wood chips or bits.

FOOD GRADE WOOD PELLETS FOR SMOKING AND GRILLING

It is important to remember that pellets of food standard and non-food grade or heating pellets are usable. Pellets for heating (or pellets used in a wood-burning furnace) may be made of wood not used for smoking meat. The taste of your food can be ruined by trees like pine or spruce. Who needs their food smelling like a car air refresher anyway? Heating pellets may also involve glues or other additives, which are not only horrible for their taste, but also awful for their wellbeing.

On the other side, pellets of food-grade wood are made solely of hardwood and do not contain any chemical binders or glues. As food use is the focus, it is produced according to the same requirements and procedures as every other foodstuff; hygiene and sanitation are at the center of manufacturing and labeling.

Since food-grade wood pellets are specifically produced for cooking, certain woods are selected because of their flavor and aroma. We'll learn what tastes are created and how they pair a little later with other products.

Food Grade Hardwood Pellets Include:

- *Mesquite*
- *Hickory*
- *Cherry*
- *Pecan*
- *Apple*

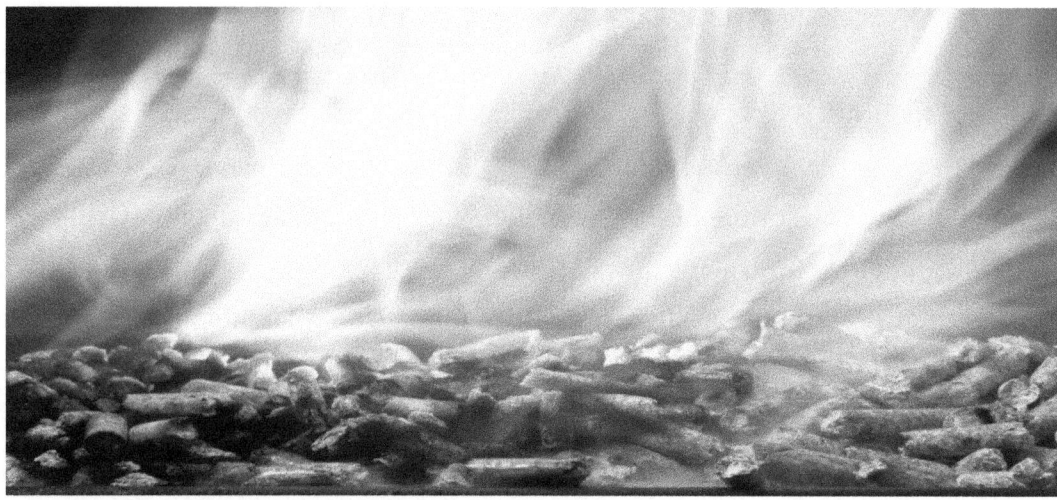

WOOD PELLETS AND THE ENVIRONMENT

You might be thinking to yourself:

"Is all that wood-burning good for the environment?"
"What about all those trees?"
"Are wood pellets better and more efficient than other fuel sources?"

These are great questions, and we are happy that you have asked them. Wood pellets originate from tree plantations (which kill the plants they are processing), storm-damaged plants, and trees in hardwood woods throughout the United States at the end of their life cycles.

WOOD PELLETS ARE PRETTY CLOSE TO BEING CARBON NEUTRAL

Trees consume radioactive carbon dioxide during their life span. The same amount of carbon dioxide is released into the atmosphere when the tree is burnt. As soon as the tree is removed, the process starts again.

LOW CO2 PRODUCTION

Including processing and shipping costs, it is calculated that the burning of wood pellets emits 34 g of carbon dioxide per kilowatt-hour of heat emitted (g / kWh). Compare that with 211 grams for gas and 64 grams for wood chips. "The Carbon Balance in Wood Fuels," Northern Woodhead, 2010.

THE BEST WOOD PELLETS FOR SMOKING AND GRILLING

If you smoke or grill a meal with a wood pellet grill, it is best to know what hardwood is needed to enhance the taste of your food.

"Should you use a pellet flavored or mixed?"

"What flavors are best for different food types?"

These are great questions when selecting pellets of wood. You do want to make sure you choose a quality pellet brand. A cheap brand can not only ruin your food but can also wreak havoc on your barbecue. That is why Louisiana Grills Wood Pellets are recommended for use on a Louisiana Grill or smoker. Because we know where they come from, we know that our goods are going to work perfectly. If you don't own a Louisiana grill, please use it as we stand firmly behind our wood pellets on other pellet grills.

WOOD PELLET TYPES

There are three kinds of pellets for smoking and grilling: flavored, mixed, and unflavored wood.

FLAVORED

Flavored pellets are made of 100% flavored wood and do not contain fillers. The tastes may vary, but Louisiana Grills produces the following kinds:

Flavor	*Description*
Tennessee Whiskey Barrel	Sweet and smoky with an aromatic tang. A premium blend of 100% oak and perfect for all your red meats.
Georgia Pecan	A very mild and nutty wood that is similar to hickory. A tremendous all-around wood that works well with poultry, beef, pork, seafood, vegetables, and cheese.
Texas Mesquite	The perfect level of bold taste to compliment your Tex-Mex cuisine. Strong aroma with a tangy and spicy flavor.
Wisconsin Hickory	Sweet with a smoky taste similar to bacon. Highly recommended for roasting your favorite meats and smoking them.
Pennsylvania Cherry	Slightly sweet with a hint of tart. Gives a rosy tint in appearance and taste to your light meats.
New England Apple	Smokey flavored with a mild sweetness. For baking, pork is strongly recommended.

BLENDED

Mixed pellets are just a mix of aromatized pellets or a mixture of aromatized and unflavored pellets. The Competition Blend Louisiana Grills includes Arable, Hickory, and Cherry.

NON-FLAVORED

Unflavored or regular wood pellets aren't desirable because of their lack of taste, but if you prefer, you can find them on the market

LOUISIANA GRILLS PELLET FLAVORS GUIDE

For all types of food, you can cook on a pellet grill or smoker, we make the perfect wooden pellet flavor. We recommend the following tastes for each type, but feel free to experiment yourself:

BEEF

Tennessee Whiskey Barrel, Georgia Pecan, Texas Mesquite, Competition Blend, Wisconsin Hickory.

POULTRY

Competition Blend, Texas Mesquite, Georgia Pecan, Wisconsin Hickory, New England Apple, Pennsylvania Cherry.

PORK

Competition Blend, Texas Mesquite, New England Apple, Wisconsin Hickory, Pennsylvania Cherry.

SEAFOOD

Competition Blend, New England Apple, Pennsylvania Cherry.

VEGGIES

Competition Blend, New England Apple, Wisconsin Hickory, Pennsylvania Cherry.

THE HISTORY OF PELLET GRILLS & SMOKERS

The hottest things in the BBQ are pellet grills — and for a good cause. Comfortable backyard cookers and friendly smokers, pellet grills cater to both beginners and pros. Simple to use, they are perfect for anyone wanting to enjoy traditional BBQ at home. Pellet grills have also become a popular smoker for many BBQers who are capable of cooking blue ribbon beef.

But the newest star of BBQ isn't all that new. The pellet barbecue has been used for almost 30 years. Over that time, it has developed into a versatile multipurpose cooker that can burn, grill, roast, and bake from an innovative alternative to conventional wood-and-coal smokers.

PELLET STOVES TO PELLET GRILLS

The roots of pellet grills (also known as pellet smokers) are traced back to the oil crisis of the 1970s and the need for an inexpensive source of fuel. One alternative was wood pellets; small hardwood capsules made from sawdust compression. By 1982, Joe Traeger, whose family owns a heating company from Oregon, began to experiment with a pellet furnace.

Pellet stoves were popular in the northwest but the name of Traeger would eventually become synonymous with another product. In 1985, during a barbecue on the fourth of July, Joe stopped cooking the chicken only to return and find the grill in flames. He kicked it in frustration and started the search for a better grill that was used to burn wood pellets.

THE BEGINNING: TRAEGER GRILLS

In 1985, Traeger produced and patented the first grill in 1986 and began manufacturing it in 1988. The external configuration of the grill was extensively taken over by conventional offset smokers — a classic drum body with a chimney. Traeger put the pellet hopper on the side of the firebox. Outside, it looked like the same smokers of charcoal and wood used for centuries. However, there was a different story inside.

Unlike pellet stoves, a simple three-position switch powered electric Traeger Grills. The wood pellets were fed into a fireplace from the hopper onto a rotating boom. A fan stoked the fire and contributed to the distribution of heat. Early Traeger Grills had to be lit manually, but the business finally began automatically with the use of ignitor rods to light up the pellets.

The food-grade pellets contain no additives except vegetable oil, often used as a lubricant during production, both for fuel source and for flavor enhancer. Pellets lit up easier than charcoal and burned cleanly because of their small size and composition. They produced in a variety of trees the smoky taste desired by lovers of the BBQ.

The Traeger Grill revolutionized smoking and made it easy and convenient. Like a gas grill, a continuous fuel source was found in Traeger Grills, which feed the pellets onto the fireplace. Without thinking about stocking coals or changing vents, you might quit. Like the conventional smoker, these grills used indirect cooking — a plate that spreads heat between the grills and the chimney, removing the flame that ruined Joe's chicken. Traeger took his reinvented Grill on the road and demonstrated to an audience that had never ever seen such a thing. Thanks to its patent, Traeger was the only name in pellet grills for 20 years and developed a loyal follow-up between BBQ lovers.

Joe sold the company in 2007, one year after Traeger's patent expired. Although the brand lived like the name in pellet grills, it now competed. Fans of Traeger Grills had their own innovative ideas.

COMPETITION ARRIVES: THE NEXT GENERATION OF PELLET GRILLS

Louisiana Grills was an early competitor who began selling grills in 2006. One of their first improvements was to put the fireplace closer to the hopper, shorten the pellets' trip and cut the pellet jams down. It's a change that brands like Memphis Wood Fire Grill and FireCraft will take later.

While Louisiana Grills has found a way for reliability to be improved, Green Mountain Grills have seen the chance to improve safety. A longstanding Traeger customer, the founder of the company, David Baker, noticed that the grills were too warm after they had been turned off, especially near the cable hopper. He replied that he designed Green Mountain Grills with a fan feature that cooled down the Grill.

"My dad's an innovator and always commented on how the grill he was grilling with could be much better," said Jason Baker, the son of David and the director of business development at Green Mountain Grills. This innovative line was obvious when it was decided to give Green Mountain Grills a peak deep deck to give roasts and turkeys more room. Other brands would use a similar concept in future years to accommodate second-hand cooking racks with more vertical space.

SET-IT AND FORGET-IT: THE EVOLUTION OF EASE

Simplicity became the starting point for the selling of pellet grills. When the truck was filled and the controller set, the Grill supplied fuel and smoke. It was a legitimate product, but had to be refined in order to compete with the best barbecues and smokers on the market.

Heat retention, particularly in cold weather, was of particular concern. "The pellet grills have not run hot enough in harsh winters," said Jeff Thiessen, President of Louisiana Grills. Even in warm weather, heat loss caused major variations in temperature that influenced cooking. One solution is thicker steel and stronger construction. Louisiana Grills took one more step, rolling metal for each grill with its corresponding plate to ensure a suitable and smooth seal.

Although better construction contributed to the efficiency of pellet grills throughout the year, temperature monitoring was the major advance. The low, medium, and high position on the initial three-position controller is approx. temperature, but in between with big jumps. Every environment was a duty cycle, the duration of the pellets fed to the auger, and then rested until they started again. However, the cycles were set. The next duty cycle was the same length when the grill had a target temperature of five or fifty degrees. Such modern grills have failed to maintain stable temperatures.

The next generation of grills included multi-position controllers with better temperature control. The sensors which read the inner temperature of the grill and provided the controller with feedback to adjust the service cycle resulted in improved accuracy. This adjustable cycle improved the precise temperature of the grills significantly.

The implementation of algorithmic technology has transformed pellet grills today into high-tech cookers with unparalleled thermal power. Such advanced grills use advanced algorithms to continuously alter the service cycle of the pellet grill, allowing them to get at the desired temperature. This has been further improved by the introduction of sporadic fans. The grill can achieve small, high-precision temperature changes by blowing short blows of air. Many companies were able to implement fully digital controllers that can be set in increments of 5°F.

Some brands have used these innovations to create smart grills to reflect the trend towards natural products. The device reads both the grill and food temperatures using a meat probe in conjunction with an internal sensor, minimizing heat when the meat is done. You will never go away so relaxed and worry-free with any outdoor cooker.

BEYOND INDIRECT GRILLING

Traditionally, smokers have done just one thing: prepare indirectly. However, modern and improved computer controllers achieve higher cooking temperatures such that some pellet grills may become flexible multifunction cookers. Grills from Louisiana, Wood Fire Grills from Memphis, Cookshack's Quick Eddy's, and FireCraft all offer the option of swapping between indirect and flame-free cooking. The same grill can now smoke a breeze, smoke a turkey, roast, or cook a pizza.

THE PLATINUM MARKET

As the grilling field grew, brands had to separate from the competition. Some have achieved so by setting up a mega premium market. These high-end units are appealing to backyard chefs and deliver sophisticated algorithmic processing, trendy looks, and superior efficiency.

"We wanted to take what had been achieved before to create differentiation," said Bob Borgerding, General Manager of Memphis Wood Fire Grills, on building a premium brand, "Their flexible stainless-steel grills touch 700°F, featuring a dual wall construction and sleek modern design. They also offer integrated options for clients who want the ultimate outdoor cooking experience. In 2016, Memphis became the first pellet grill manufacturer to include cloud-based Wi-Fi with their grills that allow users to control their grill anywhere with their phones or tablets. It was an incredible move forward for pellets and barbecues. It also resets the bar for every other producer of pellet grill, many of whom strive to adopt wireless capabilities. In reality, Wi-Fi connectivity would likely be normal in most quality pellet grills in the next few years

Quick Eddy's by Cookshack is another super-premium brand that makes wide double-wall stainless steel grills that feature sturdy, commercial exterior and flexible four-zone cooking, including areas for direct and indirect cooking and cold smoking.

THE NEW CLASS

Although new customers were drawn by the introduction of high-end grills, it also generated a gap. Traeger models were admirably good, but they missed luxury features. The ultra-luxury ones are even more costly. There was nothing in the interim.

Some companies began producing pellet grills to fill this room, which provides excellent construction and efficiency but costs less than $1,000. Firecraft manufactures a pellet grill of stainless steel, while Louisiana Grills sells several models with high duty. Both provide the newest automated controls, a meat temperature monitor, and direct cooking options to be set at a 5°F rise.

THE FUTURE OF PELLET GRILLS

Owing to the success of kitchen shows and design visiting restaurants, BBQ and barbecue are at the center of culinary culture. Pellet grills are flexible and simple to use, suitable for free movements like hot dogs and hamburgers. As a true commodity, they are perfect for people who are looking for authentic BBQ flavors but lack the resources and expertise for conventional smoking. Pellet Grills often earn fanfare on the professional circuit, with extreme smokers allowing BBQ championship.

Pellet grills in the BBQ category are the fastest growing. But they still account for only a small percentage of total grill sales. An ongoing obstacle is educating the public, most of whom do not know what to do with pellet grills.

"There's a total lack of understanding," said Jeff Thiessen. The only approach to attract clients is to display pellet grills in practice. "The show and word of mouth markets the grill — this is a local business."

The rapid rise of trademarks in large-scale shops has brought a greater market to pellet grills than ever before. This is a trend that helps any manufacturer — the more customers know about pellet grills, the more apt they are to check out what each company has to sell.

"Large development is a challenge as it arrives, not an issue," Bob Borgerding said. "Education is all about converting, and the industry needs to work together to do so."

THE REBIRTH OF TRAEGER

In 2014, Traeger was bought over by a consortium headed by former CEO of Skullcandy, Jeremy Andrus. The new company offered Traeger knowledge of marketing and skills that were not seen in pellet grills or BBQs, as well as a desire to reach the public. Traeger started to reinvent itself almost instantly, seeking a wealthier, more outgoing market. It has established a significant social media presence, has hired a gastronomic chef to create Traeger-based recipes that attract the community, and has engaged brand supporters who reflect an active, outgoing way of living. They have also updated and redesigned their grills to reflect new technological and performance advances in grill pellets.

But Traeger was not happy with marketing even the population Skullcandy he understood so well. The main aim was to make Traeger a household name, and therefore the new owners should place their grills in big box stores, where they could see the regular shopper. They also launched a Traeger Roadshow introducing the Grill and its ability to clients who could see and experience the Grill and sample the food that arrived. The local presentations were a page out of the Traeger family textbook as Joe's sons brought the first Traeger Grill across the northwest and winning over one trip at a time converts.

Recognizing that pellet grills are a show-me commodity, Traeger has been seen on the TV, delivering a half-hour newsletter that exposes millions of audiences to pellet grills and what they are capable of. Pellet grill makers knew for a better part of a decade that when people saw their grills, they would be sold. Traeger proved them right. They proved right. By the end of 2016, Traeger's marketing campaigns had become more involved in a pellet grill than ever before. For those who question the Traeger influence, consider: more than 3X were searched for the term Traeger grill as often as the term pellet grill.

The success of Traeger had a positive effect on the entire industry. Their publicity has generated a trickle-down: the more people know about Traeger, the more they are conscious about other grills. Everybody has reaped the benefits. Although Traeger has defined itself as the weber of pellet grills, which people recognize and trust, every other has been introduced to potential consumers more successfully.

HOW DOES A PELLET SMOKER WORK?

A pellet smoker operates by heating an oven, where air circulates and food is cooked by convection. Charcoal and hardwood pellets burn at the bottom of the cooking room (sometimes known as a burn pot or firepot), and food is on grills near the top of the room. When fuel is small, a pellet hopper is supplied with more wood above the cooking area. An auger drives the pellets down into the center of the room.

The airflow regulates the temperature settings for a pellet smoker. To raise temperatures, heavy-duty fans at the base of the device draw air into the lower portion of the cooking area, where the smoldering pellets absorb oxygen. Meanwhile, while the top deck is raised, heat will escape from the smoker.

HOW TO USE A PELLET SMOKER TO SMOKE MEAT

With a little practice, using a pellet grill is comfortable.

There are a few basic tips for any potential pit boss:

1. Keep cool the smoker. A big advantage of wood pellets cooking is that they fire cleanly. Don't cancel this privilege by making your grill collect burnt garbage. Following through cooking session, take some time to extract unused pellets from the hopper and clear grilled grills.

2. Using the sample temperature. Many pellet smokers today come with a meat sample, but it may be one of the lowest quality components in the entire system. Invest in a high-quality digital thermometer and be precise about cooking at the temperature you want.

3. Trial on hardwoods. You can develop your custom hardwood blend in addition to developing a custom dry rub or wet brine. You can be a purist and never combine one form of wood with another. Or perhaps you will succeed with base-wood pellets such as hickory, alder, or mesquite, and then add fruit wood pellets such as apple or cherry. Beef smokes well with all the woods except apples in general. Pork tastes good with all but oak and maple burned. When smoked with alder, maple, or mesquite, the fish

is especially delicious. When cooked on hickory, pecan, and maple wood, Vegetables can taste fantastic. Yet pork fits for just all but blended yet wood.

4. Give yourself plenty of room for cooking. If your smoker does not want his patio crowded, ensure that you have one with a fairly wide cooking area to be able to prepare your meat correctly. The best pellet grill will range from just over 200 m2 to over 800 m2, but think of your goals and pick accordingly. It is best if you have a grill a little too large instead of too small, although some circumstances (such as tailgating) do involve a smaller barbecue.

5. Carry a sear shell. Pellet smokers don't get about as heavy as regular BBQs. When you are searching for a specific appliance that can cope with both conventional pellet smoking and searing, imagine getting a pellet grill with an add-on sear box — a relatively tiny barbecue that can achieve temperatures much higher than the smoker.

ADVANTAGES OF WOOD PELLET SMOKER AND GRILLS

Food patterns and cooking methods rely on geographical locations and customs that people around the world practice. The cooking method has grown a lot over time. Many taste and spice tests have driven experienced chefs to create several delicious recipes.

Grilling and roasting are two cooking methods that give the meat a unique taste. Grilling is also a safer cooking process as it helps to retain food's nutrition and taste. The industry is bursting with grilling and roasting equipment choices. Still, selecting the right can be very challenging. This chapter offers you some of the advantages of wood pellet grills to understand why they are the best.

As you may know, many traditional types of equipment used to barbecue or to cook open fire meat use charcoal as its heat. Such conventional cooking methods create a lot of smoke, but they certainly enhance the taste and aroma.

On the other side, a wood fire pellet grill lets you quickly and smoothly grill food. It's like a convection oven that equally cooks rice. In addition, pellets and smokers are superior to traditional grilling options as they provide less acrid smoke than conventional granules and smokers. The following points address the potential benefits of wood pellet grills.

VERSATILE

Forest fire pellet grills and smokers are both thrilling with their flexibility. This ensures that you can have a selection of lip-smack food ready in minutes. Pellet grills can be used to cook all kinds of food; from chicken wings to short ribs braised.

FAST

Everything that saves time and energy should be embraced warmly. The concept of cooking food with wood pellet grills and smokers is gaining tremendous popularity. This is because these grills help people to cook food more quickly and easily. Such wood pellets grills and smokers easily preheat and save a lot of time.

BETTER TEMPERATURE REGULATION

One of the many advantages of using a wood fire grill is that it offers better ways of monitoring heat in the chamber. For conventional grills, handling the fluctuating temperature may be difficult. The proper cooking of meat demands that the temperature must be maintained under check so that the beef can retain its optimum taste.

EVEN COOKING

New wood pellet grills and smokers provide great methods of cooking food efficiently without too much trouble. Such electronic devices work to have faster and simpler grilling choices. Furthermore, pellets produced from the wood fire have a heat diffuser plate on which you can put soaked wood chips or hardwood pieces to enhance the smoke effect.

VARIETY

Cooking specialists recommend using grills and smokers with wood pellets as they come in a range of shapes and sizes. Grills and smokers are built with the needs and preferences of all kinds of customers looking for practical cooking tools in mind. The grilled pellets and smokers are sold in different varieties, including hickory, cherry, apple, and pecan.

COLD SMOKERS

In addition to wood-pellet grills, several businesses sell cold smokers. Such cold smokers are used to roast meat and salmon.

TOP 5 FEATURES SHOULD KNOW BEFORE BUYING PELLET SMOKERS

With more pellet smokers on the road, producers aim to distinguish and stand out from their rivals by establishing a high standard in the industry. They focus on improving pellet grill features that provide customers with the best benefits, satisfying their needs and expectations with advanced abilities and innovative technology.

1. PRECISE MEAT PROBES CONTROL BOARDS

Pellet grill controllers have meat-probe inputs and outputs. What you have to do is attach one end to the control board and put the other end into the product. Tracking the internal food temperature at a glance on the automated monitor without raising the plate. Not every pellet smoker has a meat sample supplied with the kit, as some of them allow you to purchase separately. Control boards are programmable and some are used for temperature regulation.

2. RELIABLE DIRECT GRILLING OPTION

With other pellet grill models, the diffuser plate has to be removed and flames can be extinguished while the permanent area is reserved with direct grilling only.

3. SPACE-SAVING SECONDARY COOKING RACKS

By purchasing a pellet grill to fit a secondary rack you will optimize your cooking space. It is important to know if the kit has an included rack or an add-on option.

4. CONNECTED WITH WI-FI CAPABILITY

You can communicate with pellet smokers as they have a Wi-Fi-fitting electronic control board. Remote controls are rendered more available through your mobile, computer, laptop, or Wi-Fi with a wired pellet smoker.

5. STATE-OF-THE-ART COOKING TECHNOLOGY

The mixture of set-it and forget-it equipment, flexibility, and taste allow pellet grills to stand out from the precision and convenience of kitchen ovens and charcoal grills. A pellet smoker can smoke, grill, roast, braise, and bake by the touch of a button and add real wood smoke to your favorite recipes.

CAN YOU USE PELLETS IN A REGULAR SMOKER?

Yeah; however, ensure that only pellets of high consistency are used without binders or glues so that they do not taste the chemicals. Never use specifically made wood pellets for home heating. Wood pellets for food may be made from a wood mixture. Some wood pellets fall down too fast while others are difficult to keep burning so that they are more suitable for shorter cooking times.

CAN YOU SOAK WOOD PELLETS?

No; pellets can improve your barbecue taste and any grilled food recipe. Pellets are easy to use, so you don't have to soak them like wood chips normally. Only 1/3 cup of hardwood pellets will provide around 30 minutes per pound of smoke.

PELLET SMOKERS BUYING TIPS

QUALITY CONSTRUCTION

The easiest way to hold your pellet smoker long is to purchase one that is well designed and features a standard design. Pellet grills don't look like offset cigarettes; they don't have to be big, but also don't have to sound fragile. To make sure that the pellet grill is sturdy, test the hardware, joints, and any welding. All seams and joints should fit in without any heat exhaust spaces or gaps.

Conduct the homework by reading feedback and analyzing the results while shopping online. Do not hesitate to ask questions or call the company's customer service. A retailer will know honestly what the basics of a pellet smoker and its relation to other versions are.

DURABILITY

When you're shopping for a pellet smoker, it is crucial to know the material it is made from. Most are made from painted steel, but the quality of steel and paint varies. A good high-temp powder coat paint withstands high heat without flaking or blistering. This is very important because steel exposure may cause rusting. Check the inside even if the outside body is painted. The diffuser plate and firepot have the potential of corroding, which is two of the most common components needing replacements. Stainless steel pellet smokers are durable, rust-resistant, and easy to maintain. The most desirable stainless steel is commercial-grade 304, and some are made of 430 stainless, which is also durable and more affordable.

TEMPERATURE RANGE

The range of temperature is essential and should match the style of cooking you expect to cook. Most have no problems hitting the correct 180°F to 425°F temperature, which is sufficient for grilling, smoking, roasting, and baking. Pallet smokers need a searing temperature of 500–550°F. Recall that a better temperature range means more types of cooking and better performance. The best-performing pellet grills range from 500°F to 700°F, which is plenty hot to provide a decent sear and tasty fire-bake pizza.

PELLET GRILL CONTROLLER

A pellet smoker should keep the temperature consistent to produce good food. The temperature will be as near as possible to 250°F for more than 12 hours; cooking is important. The efficiency of your pellet grill is strongly decided by the pellet smoker brain control panel. Pellet grill controls have multiple styles of differing quality and accuracy. The majority of pellet grills will maintain their temperature constant and reliable in optimal environmental conditions. But not all pellets can keep the temperature stable when the temperature is cold, windy, and raining.

SIZE AND COOKING AREA

Pellet smokers for a range of uses, from small pellet grills for tailgating to extra-large industrial ones, and built-in pellet smokers for open kitchens are available in many types. When it comes to barbecue scale, consider a BBQ area that suits your grill room and lifestyle. The two cooking areas of a pellet smoker comprise the main cooking area, the principal barbecue, and the whole secondary cooking field.

Since pellet grills are indirect, the main rack or the top rack will not have to be cooked as the temperature is similar — a smaller pellet smoker with a primary grid of 450 m2. and a 125 sq. in the top cabinet. This is better than a larger grill with only 500 square meters. Remember that a more popular room is not always a superior option. A pellet smoker with a primary smoking area of 450 to 500 sq. inches for a typical household. It should be time. Couples and people should go smaller, while larger families and visitors routinely will opt for bigger grills.

DIFFERENCE BETWEEN PELLET AND THE OTHER GRILLS TYPES EXPLAINED

CHARCOAL

The charcoal grill is a classic and favorite of purists; also referred to as one of the best or authentic grilling choices. Although they come in all forms and sizes, all use briquettes (sometimes mixed with wood chips) or lumps as a source of fuel that produces a distinct, long-lasting, and smoky flavor.

Cooking with charcoal is also an inherently slower way of doing cooking. Regulation of the interior temperature of the grill is more complex and less accurate and up to cooking temperatures can take up to 20 minutes for a barbecue. The clean-up is a bit tedious as well. Nevertheless, the flavor is worth the extra effort.

Charcoal grills are usually fairly cheap, from just 30 dollars up to 300 dollars. They even come in different styles:

- An open-style grill you often see in parks is a brazier grill.

- Kettle grills are standard circular grills (sometimes square) on a tripod (usually with two wheels) and a lid. Also, they have a basic vent to regulate the internal temperature.

- Yeah, a barrel grill is built like a barrel. The first models were constructed of a tank of 55 gallons turned on its side and split in two lengthwise. Remove the ring, the hinge, the bottom grate to carry the charcoal, the upper grate to cook, and some hands, and you have a barrel grill. You can, of course, buy ready-made barrel grills today.

- Cart grills are the style you usually see these days sitting outside hardware stores, but only a few of them are charcoal. Most grills in the cart-style are gas-fired grills.

- The Kamado grills are crafted from a Japanese rice cooker named a mushikamado. It is identical in form to a kettle grill but is typically a more bottomless tank, constructed of ceramic rather than metal. This insulates fire, allowing a more consistent cooking temperature throughout, and more effectively burning the charcoal. They're also tall, bulky, and very pricey with an entry-level price of around $500.

- Typically, portable grills are shorter versions of kettles, which can be packed and taken easily for a picnic or a weekend in the woods.

GAS

The other type of grilling is a gas grill. They usually come in the form factor of a cart or are installed into a permanent outdoor cooking area with a varying number of burners.

The old debate used to be between coal and gas, but now there is a new debate: natural gas or liquid propane. Natural gas burns better, it's easier to use (from half to one-sixth of the price), and no longer runs out or has to change tanks halfway through cooking. That said, with natural gas, your Grill will become a permanent facility. You're not going to be able to move it around at will.

Liquid propane is still more commonly used and adds portability convenience. But you're also going to have to plan ahead or make any rough estimates to determine how much cooking time you've left on the current tank. Luckily, if you have a gas connection in your house, you may be able to purchase a conversion kit for your existing Grill, or you may be able to enjoy both types of fuel.

The benefit of gas grills is the ease to use and accuracy. It doesn't take 20 minutes to fire a gas grill; just turn on the gas, press the igniter, and wait until it reaches the desired internal temperature. And if the grill cooks too cold or hot, just adjust the dial. Cleaning and repairs are much better on gas grills, too, without spilling any ashes. Although, you're going to miss out on that smoky taste (unless you get a smoker's box).

While there are countless models to choose from with a handful of nifty features (such as side burners or rotisserie spit), the initial decision you'll have to make when buying a gas grill is how many burners you'll need. Gas grills generally start at around $90 for two burners but can go up to $ 1,000 and up to four to six-burner grills.

ELECTRIC

Generally, electric grills are more compact and can be used both inside and outside. Think of George Foreman's grills, but there are hundreds of various types and form influences — table, foundation, pot, face open, cart, etc. A flat-top grid without a lid is one of the newest electric grill options available.

The easiest way to start grilling is by plugging it into a nearby outlet and turning your control push button. However, as you would imagine, they can only step up to their power line. If you don't have a handy outlet in the backyard, you'll need to move the barbecue or use an extension cord to power the grill.

Electric grills are frequently excellent alternatives for apartment residents who cannot cook on their balcony with (or even store) a gas or carbon grill.

Like gas grills, they lack the smoked aroma of cooking with charcoal but are a convenient and affordable way to cook that gets better over time. Grills begin at approximately $50 and can cost up to $600 for higher models.

PELLET

Pellet grills have been popular for over 30 years, but over the last couple of years, they have seen a revival. They can act as grill or smoker.

There is a pellet grill on the barbecue leg, which you can fill with pellets of food-grade material. Then toggle the control switch on and set a temperature to fire. An auger connects the hopper to a burning pot under the cooking grill and moves the pellets into a burn pot when it rotates.

The BBQ also has a so-called "oven pin" inside which the pellets fire as they fall into the burning bowl. The wood pellets burn and smoke, giving you the smoked taste of hardwood. You can cook on high flame, which is similar to other grills on the market, or make it cool and easy.

Since a computer controls a fan to store the fire and to add wood pellets to a burning pot, you must have a power source in the immediate vicinity to use a pellet grill. And you will have ashes to clean up with any use, much like a barbecue grill.

Pellet grills are usually not found in barrels or cart-type factors, although variations to the rule remain. Prices can vary from approximately $350 to $1,300.

INFRARED

Infrared grills resemble any other gas grill cart-style. They are typically operated by natural gas or liquid propane but may be electric as well. The distinction lies in how they are heating.

Instead of utilizing radiant heat by heating the air within the Barbecue, they use an electrical or gas device to heat a solid surface, such as ceramic, which emits infrared waves to heat the cooking. What you get is a heating grill that is ready to go in only a few minutes, which cooks consistently without any flare-ups.

Infrared grilling is fast; not to mention, they are also willing to exceed 700°F temperatures.

The real drawback is the size. Although infrared grills at the entry-level have come down to around $800, the overwhelming majority are setting you back $1,500 and more. That said, more infrared options are starting to hit the market, like a smoke-free indoor grill from Philips Avance.

CHOOSING THE RIGHT TYPE OF GRILL

In the end, there's no one-size-fits-all solution for too many choices on the market. Choosing the Grill for your needs would depend on what you're preparing for, the comfort you're searching for, your budget, and also where you stay.

When you're on a small schedule, infrared is automatically out. Charcoal is more difficult to use over time as it needs to remove the briquettes for increasing use. For long-term use and entry-level pricing, electric or gas is your best budget option. And for the least amount of cleaning, they are the most trouble-free.

Charcoal and pellet grills are widely agreed as the best choices for taste, but they do need more maintenance and higher operating costs. Oh, you'll need some time to make your Grill hot enough to start cooking. You're having essentially a two-in-one package with a barbecue and a smoker with a pellet stove.

It's also a perfect excuse to get your usual six-pack, a massive slab of steak, whichever Grill you want, and invite a group of buddies over to "try stuff out."

WOOD PELLET SMOKER AND GRILL RECIPES

1. TRAEGER BAKED CORN DOG BITES

PREP TIME: 15 Minutes

COOK TIME: 30 Minutes

SERVES: 10 - 12 People

Poppable, sharable, and a perfect fresh appetizer. Sweet & savory cornbread dough is wrapped around bite-sized hot dogs before being baked on the Traeger to golden perfection.

Ingredients:

- *1 cup milk, room temperature*
- *4 teaspoon active dry yeast*
- *¼ cup granulated sugar*
- *2 cup all-purpose flour*
- *1/2 cup yellow cornmeal*
- *1 teaspoon baking soda*
- *1/2 teaspoon mustard powder*
- *1/4 cup vegetable oil*
- *1/2 teaspoon cayenne pepper*
- *1 Tablespoon plus 1 teaspoon kosher salt*

- *15 cocktail beef frankfurters*
- *1 egg, lightly beaten*
- *1 teaspoon dried minced garlic*
- *Ketchup and mustard, for serving*

Steps:

1. In a bowl, combine the butter, yeast, and sugar. Set aside for 5 minutes, or until foaming starts.
2. Add flour, cornmeal, baking soda, mustard powder, butter, cayenne pepper, and a tablespoon salt.
3. Mix with a spoon, then knead into a dough with your fingertips.
4. Move the dough to a bowl and cover with plastic wrap until the dough grows and doubles in size and set aside for about 45 minutes.
5. Set the Traeger temperature to 375°F and preheat until ready to cook, and the lid is closed for 15 minutes.
6. Take dough out of the bowl and break it into 15 parts.
7. Use a rolling pin to cut each piece of dough out into 3" x 3" parts on a work surface dusted with flour.
8. Through each hot dog right in the middle of the dough board. To produce 15 mini corn dog bites, roll it in the dough and push the edges to seal.
9. Move corn dog bites to a parchment paper lined baking sheet and spray each bite gently with a beaten egg. Sprinkle with dried minced garlic and remaining salt on every slice.
10. Put sheet tray directly on the grill and bake for around 30 minutes until golden brown.
11. Serve with your choice of ketchup and mustard, or dipping sauce. Enjoy it!

2. BBQ BROWN SUGAR BACON BITES

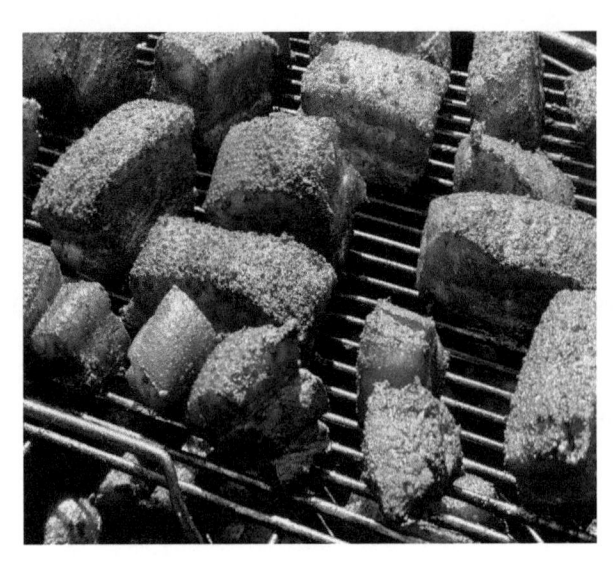

PREP TIME: 10 Minutes

COOK TIME: 25 Minutes

SERVES: 2 - 4 People

With bacon, everything's easier and that's perfect for your holiday appetizers. This unique and easy-to-make BBQ Bacon Bites recipe will become a tradition in no time.

Ingredients:

- *1/2 cup brown sugar*
- *1 Tablespoon Fennel, ground*
- *2 teaspoon kosher salt*
- *1 teaspoon ground black pepper*
- *1 Pound Pork Belly, diced*

Steps:

1. Fold an aluminum foil measuring 12" x 36" in half and crimp the bottom so it has a surface. Make a hole in the bottom of the foil using a fork. That should make some of the bacon fat clear and the bacon bites crisp.

2. Set temperature to 350°F when preparing to cook and preheat, lid shut for 15 minutes.

3. Combine brown sugar, ground fennel, salt and black pepper in a wide pot.

4. Place the sliced pork in the mixture and swirl it away. Move the pork bits to the foil.

5. Place on the grill and roast for 20-30 minutes before the bits are crispy, glazed, and bubble.

3. SMOKED BEER CHEESE DIP

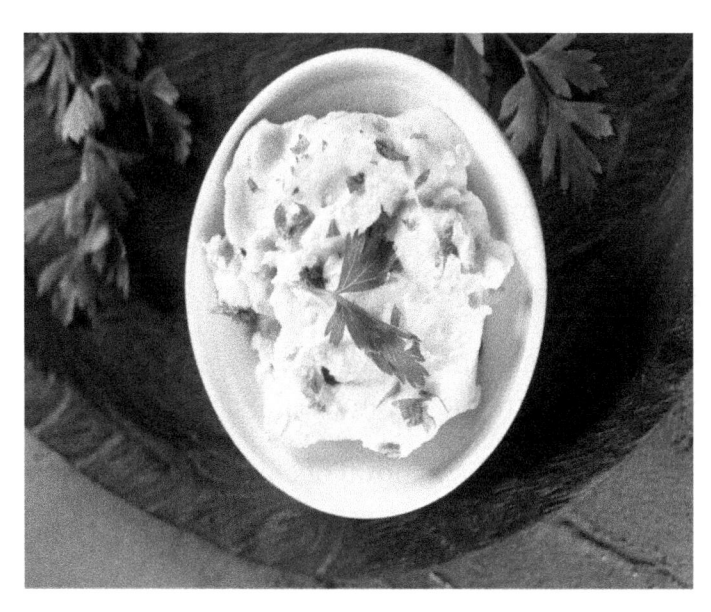

PREP TIME: 15 Minutes

COOK TIME: 1 Hour

SERVES: 6 - 8 People

Set this crispy bowl of beer-infused soup down with mates for a warm-bellied dinner.

Ingredients:

- *1 Whole Cheese, sharp cheddar*
- *1 Bottle Pale Ale Beer*
- *8 Tablespoons butter*
- *1/2 cup Baby Carrots, chopped*
- *1 Small onion, chopped*
- *3/4 cup flour*
- *1 cup heavy cream*
- *1 teaspoon Worcestershire sauce*
- *5 Dash Frank's RedHot Sauce*

Steps

1. Set the grill temperature to 180°F and preheat for 15 minutes when ready for cooking.

2. Put ice in a large pot; cover with a cooling rack and put the cheese block above. Take a big pan and pour in beer. Once the grill is fine, place the two pots on the grill and smoke for 30 minutes.

3. Remove all saucepans off the grill; cover the cheese instantly and put in the freezer to easily firm the cheese.

4. On the stovetop, heat the butter; add the carrots and the onion. Switch the stovetop heat to medium-high and simmer until the vegetables soften up and caramelize for 15 minutes. Once the veggies have been baked, add meal.

5. Stir in flavored malt, heavy cream, Worcestershire and spicy blend. Reduce to medium-low heat and simmer the liquid mixture for 15 minutes.

6. Take out from the fridge and crumble cheese. Add a handful of cheese to the stovetop to guarantee that the cheese is blended before inserting the next one. Salt and pepper to taste once all the cheese is applied.

7. Serve with heavy cream, shredded cheese and bacon soup. Serve.

4. ROASTED TINGLE WINGS

PREP TIME: 10 Minutes

COOK TIME: 30 Minutes

SERVES: 6 - 8 People

Pleasant wings of devilish seasoning. These wings are marinated with a sweet and spicy sauce and grilled fast and easily for an intense taste.

Ingredients:

- *3 Whole jalapeño*
- *1 Tablespoon Red Devil Cayenne Pepper Sauce*
- *1/2 cup Traeger Texas Spicy BBQ Sauce*
- *2 Tablespoons Traeger Blackened Saskatchewan Rub*
- *1/2 cup honey*
- *1 Tablespoon Worcestershire sauce*
- *1/4 cup water*

Steps:

1. For the sauce, add all the ingredients in a blender except the wings and mix.
2. Place the sauce into a resealable plastic bag and place the wings in the container. Marinate overnight for 1 hour.
3. Set temperature to 350°F when preparing to cook and preheat, lid closed for 10 to 15 minutes.
4. Put the wings directly on the grill and cook for 30 minutes, or until the wings are 165°F internal.

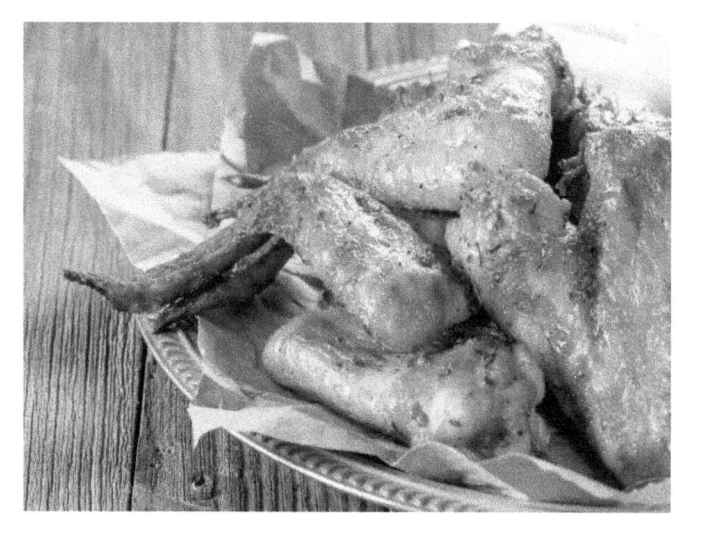

5. THE DAN PATRICK SHOW GRILLED BLOODY MARY WINGS

PREP TIME: 20 Minutes

COOK TIME: 1 Hour

SERVES: 6 - 8 People

The wings of Dan Patrick should get the audience of your game day flooding your seat. Seasoned with cocktail salt from Bloody Mary and poured into Traeger's Bloody Mary combination, these wings will blast away all the taste buds.

Ingredients:

- *2 Pound chicken wings*
- *3 Tablespoon Traeger Bloody Mary Cocktail Salt*
- *2 cup Traeger Smoked Bloody Mary Mix*

Steps:

1. Set the Traeger at 350°F when ready to cook and preheat, lid closed for 15 minutes.
2. The Bloody Mary cocktail salt wings uniformly for the season and directly on the fire. Cook for 30 minutes, until transforming into crispy and golden wings.
3. Switch the Barbecue wings to an aluminum pot and dump in the Charred Bloody Mary Blend.
4. Cover and bring back on the fire, turning halfway for another 30 minutes. Apply a little liquid to the pot if it becomes dry.
5. Move wings to a tray or board.

6. GRILLED SHRIMP TACOS WITH GARLIC CILANTRO LIME SLAW

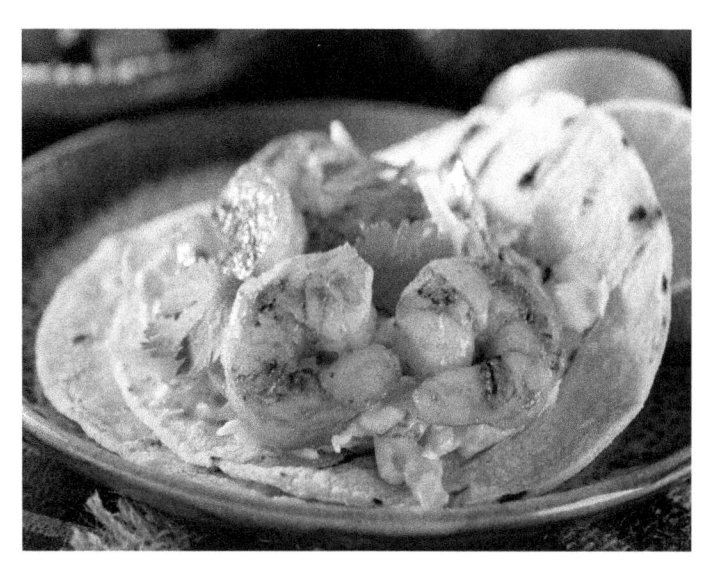

PREP TIME: 20 Minutes

COOK TIME: 8 Minutes

SERVES: 4 - 6 People

Say hello to these healthy shrimp tacos, unlike any other under the sun.

Ingredients:

- *1/4 cup olive oil*
- *1/4 cup water*
- *1/4 cup Oregano, chopped*
- *1/2 cup cilantro leaves*
- *3 Clove garlic*
- *1/2 Jacobsen Salt Co. Pure Kosher Sea Salt*
- *2 lime, juiced*
- *1/2 cup Yogurt, Greek*
- *1 Pound Shrimp, raw, peeled, deveined*
- *1 teaspoon chili powder*
- *1 teaspoon ground cumin*
- *1 teaspoon Jacobsen Salt Co. Pure Kosher Sea Salt*

- *1/4 teaspoon ground cayenne pepper*
- *3 cup Cabbage, shredded*
- *8 Small corn tortillas*
- *2 Avocado, Sliced*
- *To Taste cilantro, chopped*
- *To Taste lime, cut into wedges*

Steps:

1. In a food processor pulse all the sauce ingredients except the Greek yogurt. When the yogurt is mostly soft, add it to mix. Taste and adjust if necessary. Set aside.

2. When ready to cook, set the grill to high and preheat, lid shut for 15 minutes.

3. Place the shrimp dry and mop them up with paper towels. Grill the shrimp for 5-8 minutes, or till the shrimp is cooked.

4. Throw some of the sauce (not all) with the chop till you like the chop. You want it to be ample oil, so the chicken is a little weighted down. Use the leftover sauce on top of the tacos or in other recettes.

5. Serve a sandwich, crush the tortillas with a spoonful of avocados, cover with a few shrimps, fill with coleslaw and end with cilantro and lime wedges.

7. BROWN SUGAR AND BACON WRAPPED LIL SMOKIES

PREP TIME: 20 Minutes

COOK TIME: 30 Minutes

SERVES: 6 - 8 People

The three basic ingredients are combined to produce a triple flavor hazard. This little appetizer packs a sweet, salty punch that you can't get enough.

Ingredients:

- *1 Pound bacon, cut in half*
- *1 Whole Cocktail Sausages, 14 oz package*
- *1/2 cup brown sugar*

Steps

1. Spread out bacon strips on a cool flat sheet. Using a rolling pin to cut out the bacon strips so they become much thicker and longer.

2. Wrap per sausage in ½ bacon strip and lock it with a toothpick. Place the bacon-wrapped sausages in a single layer and top with brown sugar in a casserole dish. Switch to the refrigerator and leave them for 30 minutes.

3. Place the grill temperature at 350°F and preheat for 10-15 minutes until ready to cook. Place the sausages on a parchment-lined cookie sheet and put the sheet on the grill directly. Cook until the bacon is crispy for 25-30 minutes. Love!

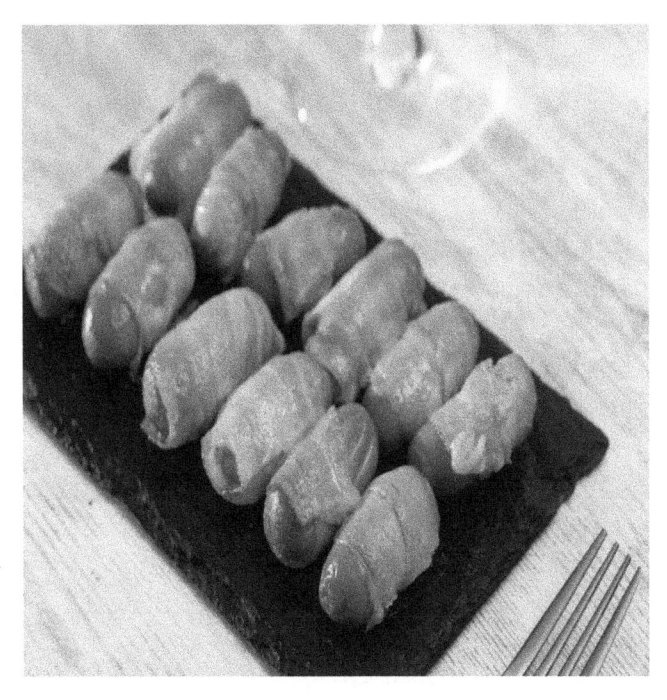

8. CHINESE JUMBO SHRIMP

PREP TIME: 1 Hour

COOK TIME: 5 Minutes

SERVES: 4 - 6 People

Put your shrimp in spicy Asian flavors, then apply a coat of tasty smoke to the wood-fired barbecue. Grilled shrimps are the perfect fast dining year-round.

Ingredients:

- *1 1/2 Pound Uncooked Shrimp, per person*
- *1 cup soy sauce*
- *1 cup Teriyaki Sauce*
- *1 cup Sweet Sherry*
- *1 cup extra-virgin olive oil*
- *1 Clove garlic, minced*
- *1 teaspoon Gingerroot, freshly grated*
- *1 teaspoon Traeger Asian BBQ Rub*

Steps:

1. Split shrimp around the back shell; cut black veins and heads of shrimps. Cover the shrimps with a moist towel of paper and put aside.
2. In a shallow pan or gallon zip-top container, add the remainder of the ingredients; blend well. Add shrimp and marinate in the refrigerator for 2 to 4 hours.
3. Set the temperature to high when ready to cook, then oil, lid closed for 10 to 15 minutes.

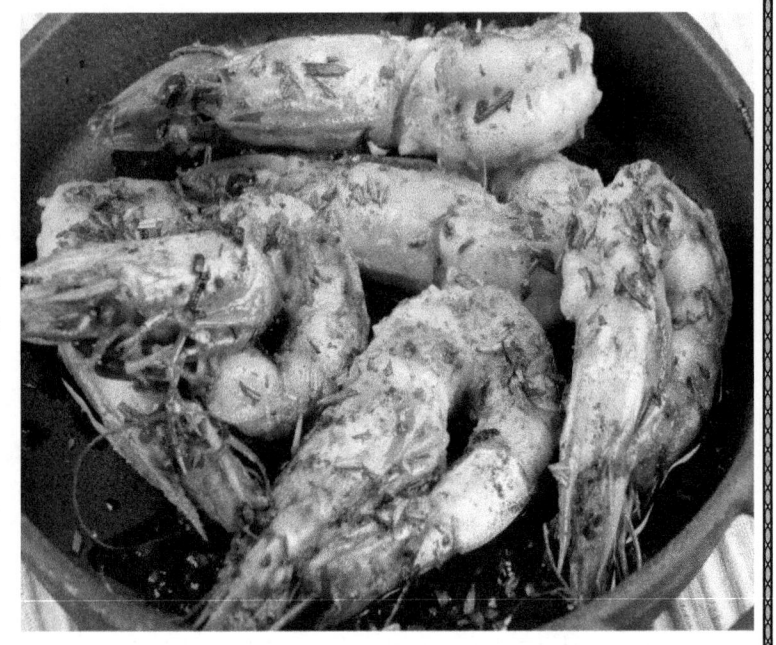

4. Drop marinade shrimp and loop on metal or pre-soaked wooden chopsticks.

5. Cover the lid and cook on the grill for 3 minutes.

6. Switch over the shrimp, shut the cover and cook for another 3 minutes or until it's opaque.

7. Remove from grill and serve as soon as possible.

9. SMOKED ALBACORE TUNA

PREP TIME: 7 Hours

COOK TIME: 4 Hours

SERVES: 4 - 6 People

New meets just that easy. A little oil, some sugar, and you have a reliable fish with any meal.

Ingredients:

- *1 cup kosher salt*
- *1 cup brown sugar*
- *Citrus Zest (1 orange or 1 lemon)*
- *6 Albacore Tuna Fillets (8 oz.)*

Steps:

1. Combine the salt, sugar, and citrus zest into a small bowl.

2. Make sure that the brine and the fish are placed in a jar, so if the fillets are lined, there is ample brine for each filet such that the individual filets do not get dry. Let stay in the fridge for 6 hours in brine.

3. take out fillets from brine and clean. Pat clear and put in the fridge for 30-40 minutes on a cooling rack.

4. Set temperature to 180°F and preheat when ready to cook, closed the lid for 15 minutes.

5. Take the fillets from the fridge and position them for around 3 hours directly on Grill grate smoking.

6. Remove from Grill and instantly enjoy, or require to cool down. It will take up to 1 week to refrigerate. Enjoy it!

10. TRAEGER SMOKED MUSHROOMS

PREP TIME: 15 Minutes

COOK TIME: 45 Minutes

SERVES: 4 - 6 People

This delicious side dish could steal the show. Mushrooms require no time to prepare and drink the rich scent of hardwood smoking. Put them into some mushroom dishes give a touch of smoke, and an earthy texture to your soup.

Ingredients:

- *4 cups Baby Portobello, whole, cleaned*
- *1 Tablespoon canola oil*
- *1 teaspoon onion powder*
- *1 teaspoon granulated garlic*
- *1 teaspoon salt*
- *1 teaspoon pepper*

Steps:

1. Blend the components together in a mixing pot.

2. Set temperature to 180°F when ready to cook, and put mushrooms on the grill and smoke for 30 minutes.

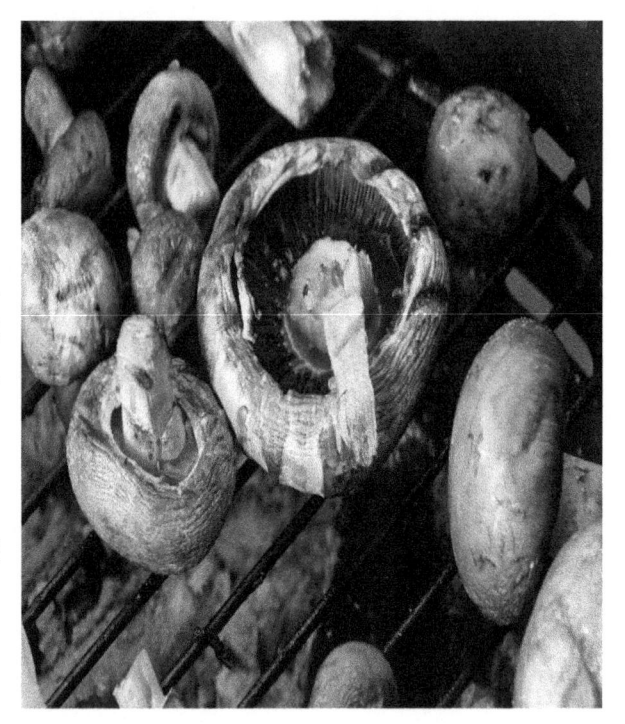

3. Boost grill temperature to high and finish cooking mushrooms, around 15 minutes longer. Serving hot. Do enjoy!

11. TRAEGER SMOKED DEVILED EGGS

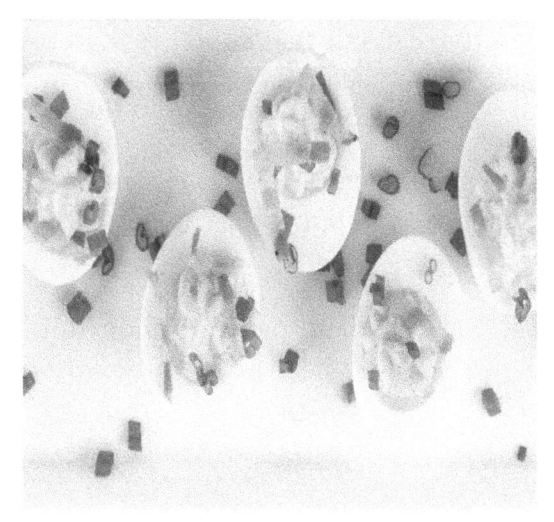

PREP TIME: 15 Minutes,

COOK TIME: 45 Minutes,

SERVES: 8 - 12 People

Whip hard-boiled egg yolks with aromatic spices and smoke them on the Traeger for a tasty holiday appetizer.

Ingredients:

- *12 Large eggs*
- *2 Whole jalapeño*
- *2 Slices bacon*
- *1/2 cup mayonnaise*
- *2 teaspoon white vinegar*
- *2 teaspoon mustard*
- *1/2 teaspoon chili powder*
- *1/2 teaspoon paprika*
- *1/4 teaspoon salt*
- *1 As Needed paprika*

- *2 Tablespoon chives, chopped*

Steps:

1. Put a big pot of water to a boil, add eggs and simmer for 9 minutes. Remove in cold water and rinse. When the eggs are cold enough to treat, cut them and break in two.

2. Set the grill temperature to 180°F and preheat when ready to cook, closed the lid for 15 minutes.

3. Put the eggs (yolk side up) on the grill and the jalapeno peppers. Cover the grill, and give 45 minutes to smoke.

4. Meanwhile, cook the bacon until it becomes crispy. Let it cool and chop until it transforms into pieces.

5. Take the eggs and jalapenos off the Traeger.

6. Slice the jalapenos on top, slice in half, remove the seeds with a spoon and dice very thin.

7. Carefully, scrape out the yolks from the eggs in a small dish. Remove the peppers with jalapeno, 1 tbsp bacon parts, mayo, sugar, butter, chili powder, paprika and oil. Using a fork, mash the mixture together and taste for seasoning. Add extra salt if necessary

8. Fill the egg white with about 2-3 tsp of the yolk mixture using either a piping bag with the largest tip or a knife.

9. Cover with a mixture of bacon and paprika pieces, and sliced chives. Enjoy it!

12. ROASTED TEQUILA-LIME WINGS BY AMANDA HAAS

PREP TIME: 15 Minutes

COOK TIME: 30 Minutes

SERVES: 6 - 8 People

These lime wings of tequila begin with a south of the rib border before a proper wood-fired roast is made. You can also pick a shot glass with a tequila-lime glaze to a taste.

Ingredients:

- *3 Pounds chicken wings*
- *2 teaspoons anchochile powder*
- *2 teaspoons brown sugar*
- *1 teaspoon granulated garlic*
- *1 taspoon cumin*
- *1 teaspoon kosher salt*
- *1 teaspoon chili powder*
- *2 Tablespoons vegetable oil*
- *1/4 cup honey*
- *1/4 cup pineapple juice*
- *3 Tablespoons Tequila*
- *1 1/2 Tablespoon hot sauce*
- *1 1/2 Tablespoon butter*

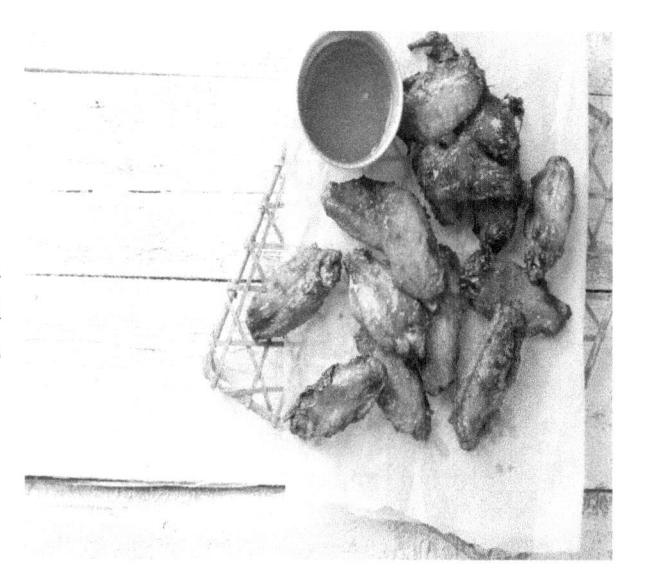

- *1 1/2 Tablespoon lime juice*

Steps:

1. Set the temperature to maximum and preheat with the lid closed for 15 minutes until ready to cook.

2. When you have bought whole chicken wings, take the tip and remove drummers and wings. Pat them dry. Remove wing tips or reserve them for storage poultry.

3. In a medium bowl, combine all the dry rub ingredients. To combine, add the oil and whisk. Remove the chicken wings and cover it.

4. For the glaze: In a small bowl, combine the ingredients of glaze. Take mild fire to a simmer. Cook until the mixture is reduced by approximately 1/3 and thicken for about 3 minutes. Keep the syrup warm while you wait for glazing.

5. Put wings directly on the grill and cook for about 20 minutes, until wings have an internal temperature of 155–160°F.

6. Brush the wings with glaze and continue cooking, around 5–10 minutes longer, before internal temperatures reach 165–175°F.

7. Eat hot. Eat nice.

13. BBQ BRISKET HOT DOG

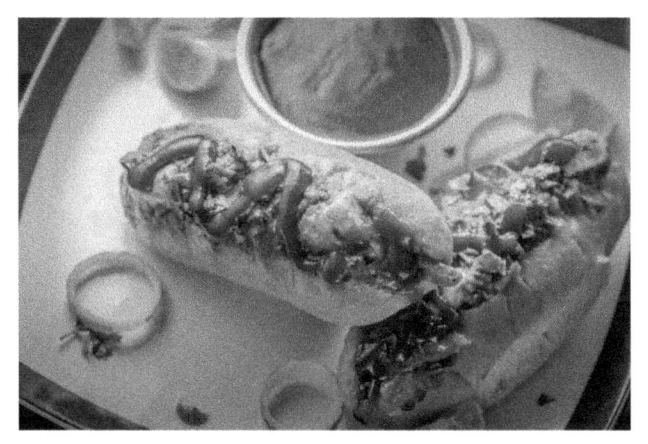

PREP TIME: 5 Minutes

COOK TIME: 10 Minutes

SERVES: 4 - 6 People

This isn't your average hot dog. Top your hot dogs with tender brisket, cheddar cheese, jalapeños and Onions, and bring them to a bold taste and complete with our BBQ sauce Sweet & Fire.

Ingredients:

- *6 Whole Hot Dogs*
- *1/2 Pound leftover beef brisket*
- *1/2 cup Traeger Sweet & Heat BBQ Sauce*
- *6 Whole hot dog buns*
- *1/2 cup shredded cheddar cheese*
- *1 onion, diced*
- *2 Whole Jalapeño, seeded and diced*

Steps:

1. Launch the Traeger with grill directions when ready to cook. Adjust the temperature to 450°F (if WiFIRE-enabled, adjust to 500°F) and close the lid for 10–15 minutes.

2. Place the hot dogs directly on the grill and cook for 7–10 minutes until slightly browned and warmed.

3. Wrap brisket pieces with a little BBQ sauce in aluminum foil to keep moist. Place directly on the grill grate next to the hot dogs and cook until warmed through, about 5–7 minutes.

4. Serve with a bun hot dog, top with brisket, additional BBQ sauce, cheddar cheese, onion and jalapeños. Enjoy!

14. GRILLED HONEY GARLIC WINGS

PREP TIME: 30 Minutes   **COOK TIME:** 1 Hour

SERVES: 6 - 8 People

The perfect mix of sweetness and some wood-fired heat. These wings are seasoned with Pork & Poultry Rub, grilled and tossed into an extra-world wing in a spicy honey garlic sauce.

Ingredients:

- *2 1/2 Pounds chicken wings*
- *As Needed Traeger Pork & Poultry Rub*
- *4 Tablespoons butter*
- *3 Clove garlic, minced*
- *1/4 cup honey*
- *1/2 cup hot sauce*
- *1 1/2 cup blue cheese or ranch dressing*

Steps:

1. Start with the wings segmented into three pieces, cutting through the joints. Discard the tips of the wing or save them from stock making.
2. Layout of the remaining pieces lined with non-stick foil or parchment paper on a rimmed baking sheet. Season well with the rubbing Traeger Pork and Poultry.
3. Set the temperature to 350°F and preheat when ready to cook, the lid closed for 15 minutes.
4. Place the baking sheet with wings directly on the grill and cook for 45–50 minutes, or until the bone is hot.
5. To make the sauce: Melt butter in a casserole. Add the garlic, then sauté 2-3 minutes. Add the honey and hot sauce, and cook until completely combined for a few minutes.
6. Keep the sauce hot while cooking the wings. Once wings are finished, pour over the wings the spicy honey-garlic sauce, turning to coat with pliers.
7. Cook the sauce for another 10–15 minutes to set.
8. Serve with ranch dressing or blue cheese. Enjoy it!

15. ROASTED ARTICHOKES WITH GARLIC BUTTER

PREP TIME: 15 Minutes

COOK TIME: 1 Hour

SERVES: 2 - 5 People

Put out the taste of fresh artichokes on the grill gradually. Drizzle for a great tasteful appetizer of homemade black garlic sauce.

Ingredients:

- *2 Large Artichokes*
- *3 Tablespoons olive oil*
- *Pinch sea salt*
- *1 Stick unsalted butter*
- *2 Clove garlic, chopped*
- *1 whole lemon halved*

Steps:

1. Set the temperature to 375°F and preheat for 15 minutes until ready to cook.
2. Meanwhile, cut off from the artichokes and throw away little outer seeds. Use a knife to slice the tops of the artichoke, and then hack off thorns on the other artichokes by using scissors. Cut the base of the stem and then peel the rough and fibrous exterior layer of the plant. Eventually, halve the artichokes and rinse clean.
3. Move the artichoke to a large bowl, drizzle with olive oil and sprinkle generously with sea salt. Toss to completely coat the artichokes. Take to the grill, cut side down and roast until the bottoms of the artichoke are soft, about 50–60 minutes when punched with a bell or knife.

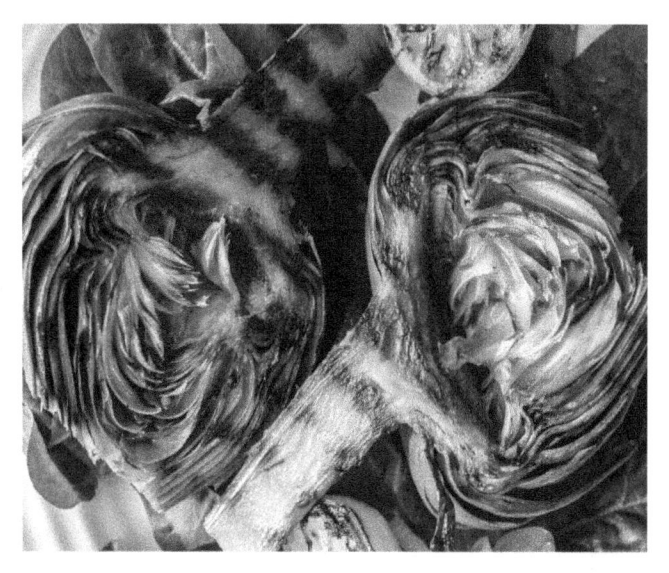

4. When the artichokes are nearly finished, add butter, chopped garlic and a pinch of sea salt to a small cup and gradually melt over medium-low heat. When the butter melts and gently bursts, introduce the herbs.

5. When the artichokes are done, move to a paper-lined bowl with the cutting sides. Clean half the garlic butter and press over the artichokes part of the lemon. Fill the artichokes with a slight sprinkling of sea salt. Serve with a ramekin of the remaining butter and extra lemon wedges. Love! Enjoy!

Chef Tip: A ramekin of healthy mayonnaise combined with a little hot sauce should also be eaten. * Cook times differ based on fixed temperatures and the environment.

16. SMOKED SHRIMP AND GRILLED DUNGENESS CRAB COCKTAIL

PREP TIME: 1 Hour

COOK TIME: 50 Minutes

SERVES: 1 - 1 People

Take a taste of this drink of seafood. Smoked shrimp and crab follow the new coriander, citrus fruit and combined with a hot clamato for a tasty wood-fired meal.

Ingredients:

- *1 Dungeness Crab*
- *1/2 cup olive oil*
- *3 Clove garlic*
- *3 Tablespoon lime juice*
- *1/4 cup cilantro*
- *1/4 Pound Shrimp, raw, peeled, deveined*

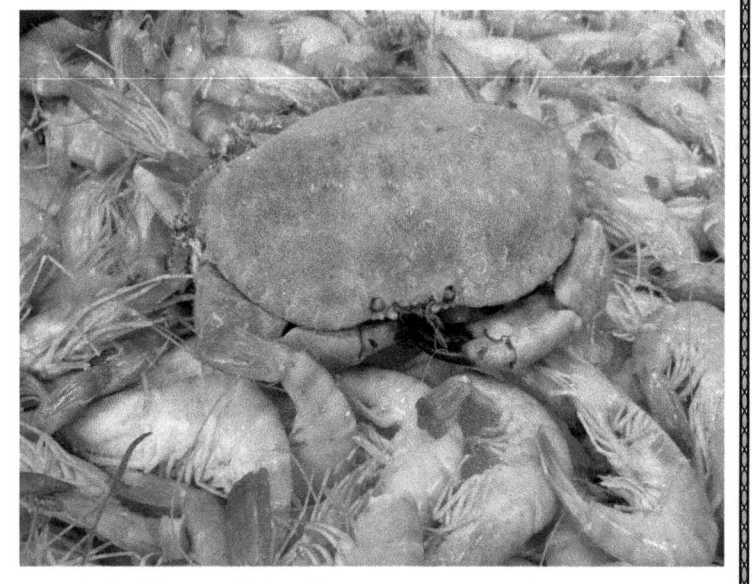

- *1 cup Clamato*
- *1/2 cup ketchup*
- *1 teaspoon hot sauce*
- *1 teaspoon salt*
- *1/2 cup onion*

Steps:

1. For crab: take the triangular tab out of the abdomen. Remove the shell. Clean indoors and crab gills, wash and rinse. Press and keep dry.
2. In a small bowl mix olive oil, garlic, 3 tbsp lime juice and 1/4 cup minced cilantro. Divide marinade between crab and shrimp for 60 minutes.
3. Set the temperature to 180°F and preheat the grill to cook for 15 minutes.
4. Put the shrimp directly on a grill and smoke, about 30–40 minutes, until firm and bronzed with smoke.
5. Remove from the grill and let it cool. Increase the grill temperature to high and preheat.
6. Place the crab on the grill grate directly. Cook the crab for 4 minutes per side until meat is opaque in the eyes. Apply often the remaining marinade to the lobster.
7. While the crab is frying, add cramato and ketchup, lime juice, hot sauce, butter, onion and cilantro in a small bowl.
8. Split the shrimp in 2/3 parts into small pieces. Remove all the crab product. Apply shrimp and crab to the cup of the cocktail and blend.
9. Put in cups and garnish with the remainder of the shrimp.

17. BBQ SPARERIBS WITH SPICY MANDARIN GLAZE

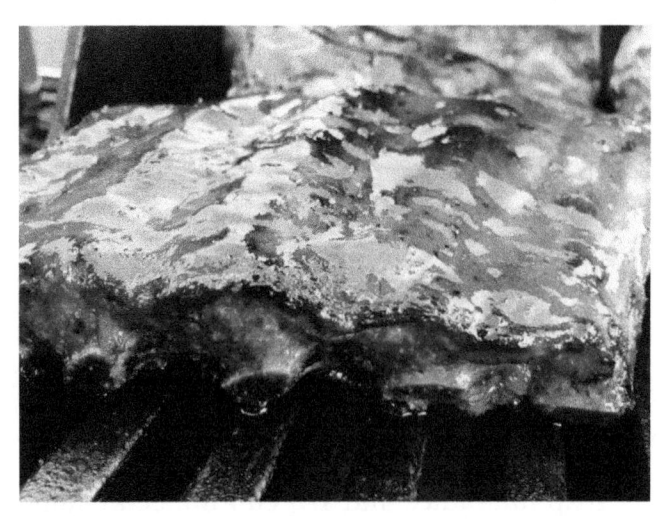

PREP TIME: 10 minutes

COOK TIME: 3 ½ hours

SERVES: 4-6 people

We added some Asian flair to the popular 3-2-1 method. These ribs have a great flavor that packs a punch of heat.

Ingredients:

- *3 Large Spare Ribs, Membrane Removed*
- *3 Tablespoons yellow mustard*
- *1 Tablespoon Worcestershire sauce*
- *1 cup honey*
- *1 1/2 cup brown sugar*
- *As Needed Traeger Pork & Poultry Rub*
- *13 Fluid Ounce Traeger Mandarin Glaze*
- *1 teaspoon sesame oil*
- *1 teaspoon soy sauce*
- *1 teaspoon garlic powder*

Steps:

1. Set the Traeger to 225°F when ready to cook, and preheat, lid closed for 15 minutes.

2. Apply the Worcestershire sauce and the mustard paste on all sides of the ribs. Put on the grill for 3 hours to smoke.

3. In aluminum foil plate, position the ribs. Sprinkle over the ribs with the brown sugar and sprinkle the Traeger Pork & Poultry. Pour over the ribs Dr. Pepper.

4. Bring the Grill to 275°F and cover with film; cook ribs for 2 hours.

5. Take the ribs out of the foil pan and turn Grill upwards. Mix Mandarin Glaze, sesame oil, soy sauce and powdered garlic. Brush the ribs and put the meat on the Traeger side for a further 8–10 minutes.

6. Serve and appreciate!

18. ROASTED BUFFALO WINGS

PREP TIME: 10 Minutes

COOK TIME: 30 Minutes

SERVES: 4 - 6 People

Of one occasion, these smoked buffalo wings are the number one crop. The spicy buffalo sauce mixes the bone wood-fired taste with the inability to deliver your Super Bowl party.

Ingredients:

- *4 Pound chicken wings*
- *1 Tablespoon corn starch*
- *As Needed Traeger Chicken Rub*
- *To Taste kosher salt*
- *1/2 cup Frank's RedHot Sauce*
- *1/4 cup spicy mustard*
- *6 Tablespoon unsalted butter*

Steps:

1. Set the Traeger temperature to 375°F when ready to cook, then preheat, lid closed for 15 minutes.

2. Dry the chicken wings with a paper towel as the grill is preheating. In a wide bowl, position the wings and sprinkle with maize, Traeger Chicken rub and salt to taste. Mix to coat the chicken wings on all ends.

3. When the grill is warm, place the wings and cook a total of 35 minutes, turning halfway through the cook.

4. Test the internal wing temperature at 35 minutes. At least 165°F should be the internal temperature. An internal temperature of 175-180°F however will produce a better texture.

5. Add the redhot souce, mustard and butter to the buffalo sauce in a saucepan. Whisk in the stovetop to combine and heat. Hold the sauce moist when frying the wings.

6. When the wings are finished, remove from the grill, place them in a medium bowl and pour the buffalo sauce over the wings and cover it with tongs.

7. Cook the wings on the grill for an additional 10–15 minutes. Serve wings dressed in ranch or blue cheese.

19. PROSCIUTTO WRAPPED DATES WITH MARCONA ALMONDS

PREP TIME: 10 Minutes

COOK TIME: 5 Minutes

SERVES: 8 - 12 People

Savory prosciutto is bundled around soft Medjool dates packed with Marcona's almonds for an appetizer full of flavor.

Ingredients:

- *24 Whole Medjool Dates*
- *1 Tub Marcona Salted Almonds*
- *8 Ounce Prosciutto Ham*
- *2 Tablespoon olive oil*
- *2 Whole Limes*
- *To Taste olive oil*
- *To Taste honey*

Steps:

1. Set the temperature to 400°F and preheat, lid closed for 15 minutes until ready to cook. Put a large cast iron pot into the barbecue to preheat.
2. Cut a break lengthways across the top of every date with a tiny paring knife.
3. Replace boxes with 1–2 marcona almonds and then press your fingers to seal the dates back.
4. Cut the prosciutto into 24 longitudinal pieces. Position one at the bottom of a strip of prosciutto to finish each date, wrap the prosciutto around the date to cover, leaving a bit of the date at each end.

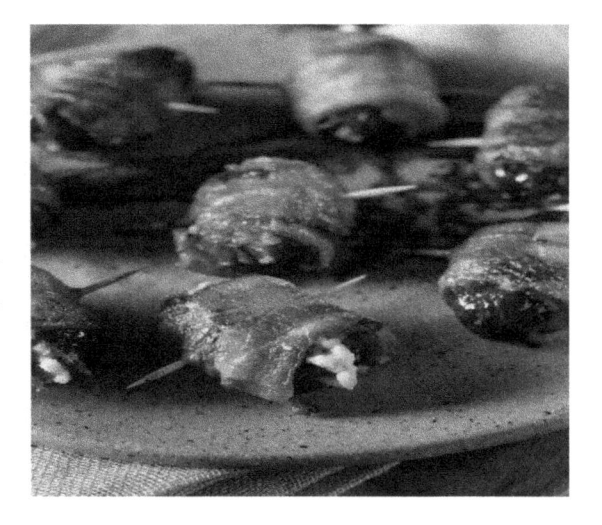

5. Add 2 tbsp olive oil to the cast iron pre-heated pot. Put the dates in the pan and cook, sew on all sides of the prosciutto and turn about 3–5 minutes total when needed.

6. When the prosciutto is uneven, detach the pot gently from the barbecue.

7. Toss the limes on the bread and add the citrus zest in the olive oil and on the dates. Put the dates on a serving dish.

8. Sprinkle with flake salt, add a flake of olive oil, sugar if you are using, and serve.

20. TEXAS PINTO BEANS BY DOUG SCHEIDING

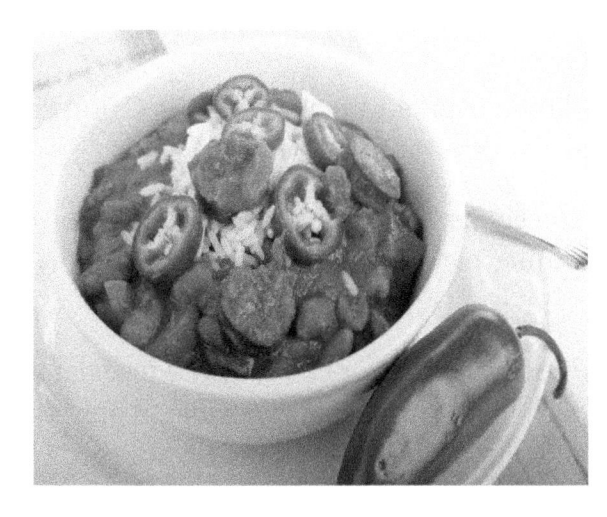

PREP TIME: 4 Hours,

COOK TIME: 6 Hours,

SERVES: 8 - 12 People

Pinto bean recipes are as preserved as brisket recipes in Texas, maybe more. These Texas Pinto Beans by Doug Scheiding are his initial competition recipes, which have always taken first place. Prepare these beans with faith in your next family or group.

Ingredients:

- *16 Ounce Pinto Beans, dried*
- *6 cup Distilled Water*
- *2 1/2 Tablespoon Tony Chareries Cajun Salt*
- *5 Pieces Black Pepper Center Cut Bacon*
- *1 Whole Medium Onion, finely chopped*
- *6 Whole garlic*
- *1/4 Pound 1/4 LB Pork Salt, Cubed in 6-8 Pieces*
- *2 Whole jalapeño*
- *2 teaspoon chili powder*
- *1 Tablespoon black pepper*
- *3 teaspoon cumin*
- *2 teaspoon Traeger Rub*
- *2 Slices White Bread*

Steps:

1. In a 5-quarter Netherland oven, drain the dry pinto beans. Cover the beans with tap water and swirl for a few minutes with your hand to avoid some dirt and dust. Drain the water.

2. Attach 6 cups of clean water to the Netherlands oven and blend with 1.5 Cajun salt tablespoons. Cover and let the beans to soak for three to four hours.

3. Cook the bacon to medium crispy on the traeger or stovetop and put it on a towel. Place the finely chopped onion in the remaining bacon grate and stir for about 5–7 minutes until translucent.

4. Smoked garlic: Set the temperature to 180°F when ready for cooking and preheat for 15 minutes. Cut off 8–10 heads of white garlic with most cloves visible. Apply raw canola oil, garlic and Cajun salt. Put garlic and smoke on the grill for 1.5 hours.

5. Switch garlic to an oven or baking tray, cover with foil, and steam for another 60 minutes. Remove the garlic and allow it to cool.

6. Increase the temperature of the grill to 350°F and preheat. For beans: detach the deck from the beans, remove any free skin and damaged or unattractive beans (only competition needs this step). Then apply all the spices (except Cajun seasoning), the salt of the hog, the onion, and two jalapeños whole. Take the cooled bacon, cut all burnt bits, and then crumble with your hands onto the skins. Finally, introduce the smoked cloves of garlic that break between the fingers as you mix the beans.

7. Place the Netherlands oven on the grill and carry to a boil. Cook 90 minutes. Swirl.

8. After 1.5 hours, cut the jalapeños, longer if you like extra oil. Reduce the grill to 325°F and start cooking beans for another 60 minutes.

9. The beans will begin at this time to become tender. Tear two slices of crustless bread into small pieces to thicken the juice into a gravel and add them to the beans. Add more bread for thicker gravy and more Tony's for salt flavor tastes if desired.

10. Stir every 10 minutes, and in 45–60 minutes, the beans should be fine.

21. STUFFED JALAPENOS

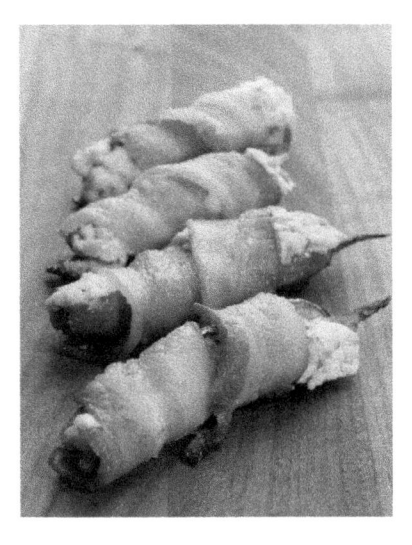

PREP TIME: 10 Minutes

COOK TIME: 1 Hour

SERVES: 8 - 12 People

Set the day on smokin 'and barbecue.' Throw these jalapeno bits on the barbecue and put them together for a burly rost during sluggish smoking. Start the taste buds with seasoning and then pursue them with the savory roasted pork. A day of traeger is memorable and full of flavor.

Ingredients:

- *40 Whole jalapeño*
- *8 Ounces cream cheese, room temperature*
- *1 cup Sharp Cheddar Grated*
- *1 1/2 teaspoon Traeger Pork & Poultry Rub*
- *2 Tablespoons sour cream*
- *1 Whole Package Mini Sausages*
- *20 Whole Slices of Smoked Bacon, Cut in Half*

Steps:

1. Wash the jalapenos and dry them. Cut the stem off using a paring knife and scrub through jalapenos with the same knife or a small metal spoon. Place Set aside.
2. Combine the sour cream, sugar, pork and poultry rub in a small bowl with savory sauce.

3. Transfer the mixture to a heavy plastic bag and cut one-half-inch off one of the bottom corners with a scissor. Squeeze in each jalapeno the cream cheese mixture, then fill them over the halfway mark.

4. Stuff in every jalapeno one sausage. Put a piece of bacon outside, securing 1 or 2 toothpicks.

5. Arrange jalapenos on a layer of paper. Start Traeger and smoke the jalapenos for 1-1/2 hours until ready to cook.

6. Boost heat to 350°F and continue to cook for 20–30 minutes or to make the bacon crispy and tangy.

22. GRILLED SHRIMP COCKTAIL

PREP TIME: 15 Minutes

COOK TIME: 10 Minutes

SERVES: 2 - 4 People

Serve this fiery cocktail of smoking shrimp on your next meal. The grilled shrimp recipe has a big flavor and is full of a spicy homemade cocktail sauce.

Ingredients:

- *2 Pounds Shrimp, tails on, deveined*
- *2 Tablespoons olive oil*
- *1 teaspoon Old Bay Seasoning*
- *1/2 cup ketchup*
- *2 Tablespoons prepared horseradish*
- *1 Tablespoon lemon juice*
- *To Taste kosher salt*

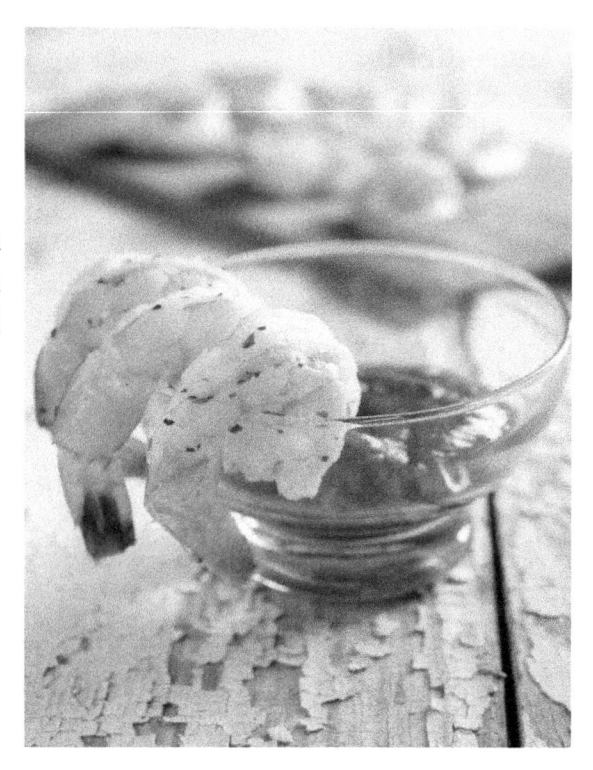

- *To Taste freshly ground black pepper*
- *Hot sauce*
- *Italian Parsley, chopped*

Steps:

1. Set the temperature to 350°F (185°C) when ready for cooking and preheat, lid closed down 15 minutes.
2. Combine the shrimp with the oil and the Old Bay seasoning in a large bowl. Add 1 tsp salt and 1/2 tsp freshly ground black pepper, unless seasoned.
3. Stir until the shrimp are well coated and place the shrimp on a grill.
4. Place the baker's sheet on the grill with the shrimp and cook for about 5–7 minutes until opaque.
5. Add ketchup, horseradish and lemon juice to the cocktail sauce. Apply the hot sauce to taste with salt and pepper if desired.
6. Serve the sauce of a drink in a cup next to the shrimp and incorporate parsley.

23. BAKED ARTICHOKE PARMESAN MUSHROOMS

PREP TIME: 15 Minutes

COOK TIME: 30 Minutes

SERVES: 8 - 12 People

Smoked champagne caps are finger foods that explode in every bite with savory flavour. You can't pop just one; smoke-infused mushroom on the barbecue is a perfect smash.

Ingredients:

- *8 Cremini Mushroom Caps*
- *6 1/2 Ounce Artichoke Hearts*
- *333/1000 cup Parmesan cheese, grated*
- *1/4 cup mayonnaise*
- *1/2 teaspoon garlic salt*
- *As Needed Your Favorite Hot Sauce*
- *As Needed paprika*

Steps:

1. Clean the mushrooms with a wet towel of paper. Remove the stems and recycle or preserve them for a later purpose.

2. Scoop off the inside with a tiny spoon (gills, etc.). Put the artichoke, parmesan, mayonnaise, garlic salt and hot sauce together and blend.

3. Mound the mushroom caps to top. Clean the paprika tips.

4. Place the mushrooms in an oven-safe bakery.

5. Set the temperature at 350°F and preheat the cover when ready for cooking for 15 minutes.

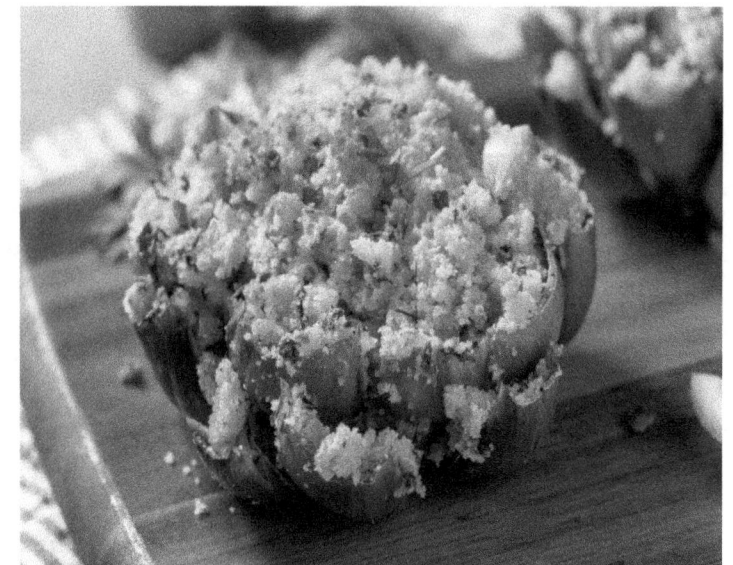

6. Bake the mushrooms (uncovered) before they bubble and start browning, about 25–30 minutes. Serve immediately.

7. Simply add your preferred bulk sausage to the mushrooms and roast on your Traeger, as led above.

24. GRILLED SWEET CAJUN WINGS

PREP TIME: 15 Minutes

COOK TIME: 30 Minutes

SERVES: 4 - 6 People

In the mood for a short and spicy snack? Smother your chicken wings in the spices of Traeger Rub and Traeger Cajun and grill.

Ingredients:

- *2 Pound chicken wings*
- *As Needed Traeger Pork & Poultry Rub*
- *Traeger Cajun Shake*

Steps:

1. Add Traeger Sweet rub and Traeger Cajun shake on the wings.
2. Set the traeger to 350°F and preheat, lid closes for 15 minutes when ready to cook.
3. Cook for 30 minutes or until the skin is dark and the center temperature test is at least 165°F with an instant-scan thermometer. Serve, yes!

25. BAKED CAULIFLOWER TOTS

PREP TIME: 20 Minutes,

COOK TIME: 15 Minutes,

SERVES: 6 - 8 People

You don't have to sacrifice taste when eating healthy. Let our signature wood-fired flavor elevate this baked cauliflower tot's recipe.

Ingredients:

- *1 teaspoon kosher salt*
- *1 Head Cauliflower, cut into florets*
- *2 eggs*
- *1/2 cup panko breadcrumbs*
- *3/4 cup cheddar cheese*
- *1/4 cup Parmesan cheese*
- *3 Tablespoons chives, chopped*
- *1/2 Tablespoon garlic powder*
- *1/2 Tablespoon onion powder*

Steps:

1. Put to a boil a big pot of salted water. Place the cauliflower blooms in the boiling water and cook until tender for 5–7 minutes.

2. Strain and put florets in an ice bath directly. Strain again when it's cold and put the florets in the food processor's tank, then rotate until the florets are like pasta. Process the florets to an even texture in batches.

3. Put cauliflower rice on a double layer and make it into a ball. Squeeze extra water (remove as many as possible) and pass cauliflower rice to a wide pot.

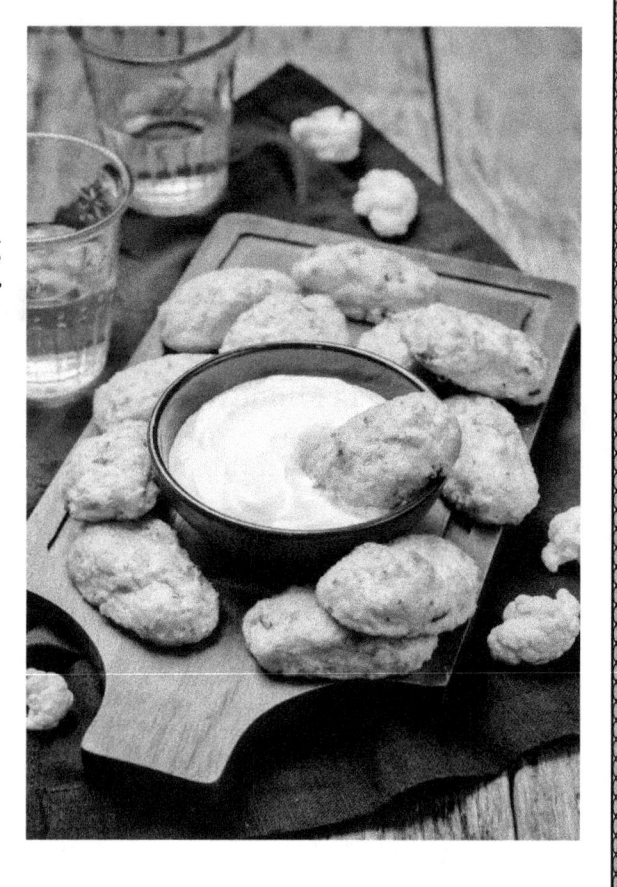

4. Add the remaining components and combine together. If the combination seems moist or cold, change the breadcrumbs with an additional egg or panko until the blend is firmer.

5. Shape the mixture into the desired form and put it on a plate tray. Take to the fridge and let the tots rest for 30 minutes (this lets them retain their form and stay together).

6. Set temperature to 375°F when ready to cook and preheat, lid shut down for 10–15 minutes.

7. Clean the grill with a grill brush and brush the grill with canola oil. Place the tots on the barbecue on the sides.

8. Cook the tots 10–15 minutes or until gently browned. Resist the tentation of moving them too far or too early.

9. To have the highest performance, take them out one by one. Serve with your own sauces for dipping.

26. WILD TURKEY SOUTHWEST EGG ROLLS BY JEREMIAH DOUGHTY

PREP TIME: 15 Minutes

COOK TIME: 40 Minutes

SERVES: 4 - 6 People

You'll go crazy to make egg rolls from this southwest. Wild turkey encounters a piece of corn, black bean and pepper, and coils into a small, crispy shell to render it beautifully unpredictable.

Ingredients:

- *As Needed extra-virgin olive oil*
- *1/2 cup White Onion, chopped*
- *1 Whole Poblano Pepper, chopped*

- *4 Clove garlic, minced*
- *1 Can Original Rotel Diced Tomatoes and Green Chilis*
- *1/2 cup Black Beans*
- *2 cup Leftover Wild Turkey Meat*
- *3 Tablespoon Taco Seasoning, dry*
- *1/3 cup water*
- *12 Whole Egg Roll Wrappers*

Steps:

1. Apply olive oil to a big pot and cook over low fire on the burner. Add the onions and peppers and sauté until soft for 2 to 3 minutes. Cook for 30 seconds, then add the garlic and black beans. Reduce heat and cook.

2. Pour over the beef, the taco seasoning, then apply 1/3 cup of water, then combine thoroughly. Add to the veggie blend and mix well. Give 2 tbsp of water if it is necessary. Cook until is ready.

3. Remove the heat and put the mixture in the refrigerator. Before stuffing the egg rolls, the mixture must be fully cooled, or the wrappers break.

4. In each wrapping, place a spoonful of the blend and seal tightly. Do the same on other wrappers.

5. Set the grill temperature strong when preparing to cook and preheat the cover closed for 15 minutes.

6. Rub with oil or butter per egg roll and place it directly in the Traeger oven. Cook for about 20 min on either side before the exterior is crispy.

7. Clear from Traeger and cool. Serve

27. FOCACCIA

PREP TIME: 25 Minutes

COOK TIME: 40 Minutes

SERVES: 4 - 6 People

It's just the beginning of herb-infused flatbread; grab two slabs, pack them with shredded pork or beef and slather with a BBQ sauce for a tasty, flavored meal.

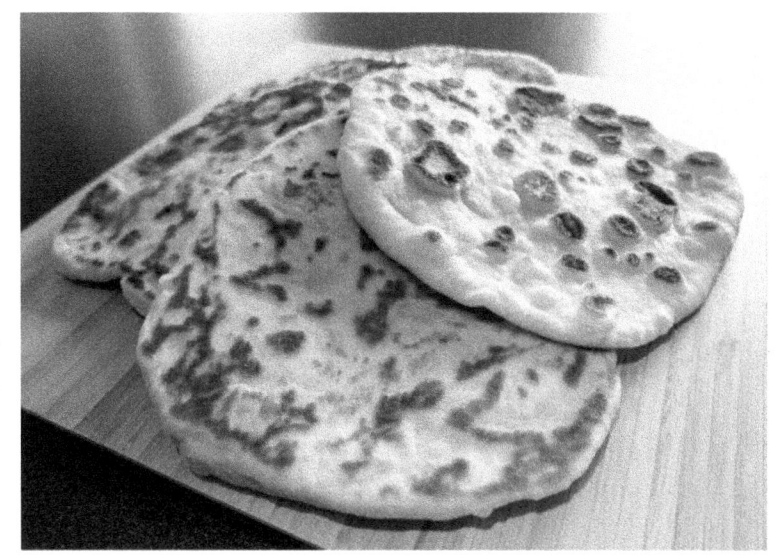

Ingredients:

- *1 cup warm water (110°F to 115°F)*
- *1/2 Ounce Yeast, active*
- *1 teaspoon sugar*
- *2 1/2 cup flour*
- *1 teaspoon salt*
- *1/4 cup extra-virgin olive oil*
- *1 1/2 teaspoon Italian herbs, dried*
- *1/8 teaspoon red pepper flakes*
- *As Needed coarse sea salt*

Steps

1. Measure the water in a glass-measuring cup. Stir in the yeast and sugar. Let rest in a warm place. After 5 to 10 minutes, the mixture should be foamy, indicating the yeast is "alive." If it does not foam, discard it and start again.

2. Pour the water/yeast mixture in the bowl of a food processor. Add 1 cup of the flour, as well as the salt and 1/4 cup of olive oil. Pulse several times to blend. Add the remaining flour, Italian herbs and hot pepper flakes.

3. Process the dough until it's smooth and elastic and pulls away from the sides of the bowl, adding small amounts of flour or water through the feed tube if the dough is respectively too wet or too dry.

4. Let the dough rise in the covered food processor bowl in a warm place until doubled in size, about 1 hour

5. Remove the dough from the food processor (it will deflate) and turn onto a lightly floured surface.

6. Oil two 8 to 9-inch round cake pans generously with olive oil. (Just pour a couple of glugs in and tilt the pan to spread the oil.) Divide the dough into two equal pieces, shape into disks, and put one in each prepared cake pan.

7. Oil the top of each disk with olive oil and dimple the dough with your fingertips. Sprinkle lightly with coarse salt, and if desired, additional dried Italian herbs.

8. Cover the focaccia dough with plastic wrap and let the dough rise in a warm place; about 45 minutes to an hour.

9. When ready to cook, start the Traeger grill and set the temperature to 400°F and preheat, lid closed, for 10 to 15 minutes.

10. Put the pans with the focaccia dough directly on the grill grate. Bake until the focaccia slices of bread are lightly golden and baked through, 35 to 40 minutes, rotating the pans halfway through the baking time.

11. Let cool slightly before removing from the pans. Cut into wedges for serving.

28. ROASTED POTATO POUTINE

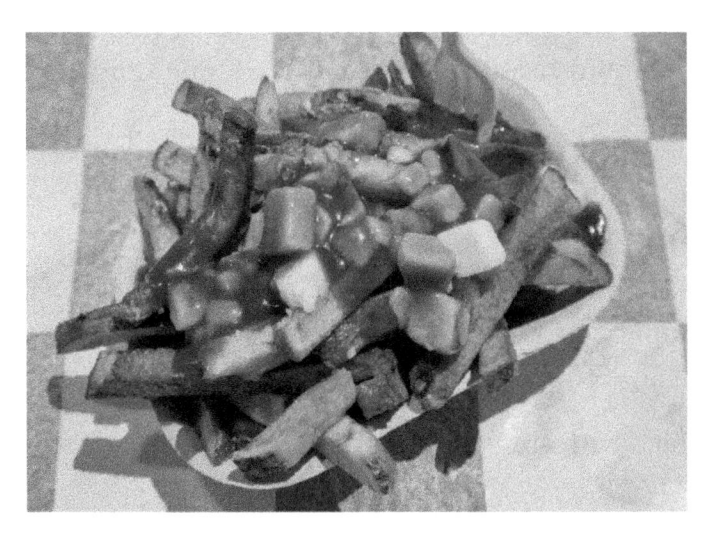

PREP TIME: 15 Minutes,

COOK TIME: 40 Minutes,

SERVES: 6 - 8 People

Roasted beans, chili, wood-fired curds, and bacon. That is beauty in appetizers. Bust this whimsical roasted potato poutine recipe for a big game or large group.

Ingredients:

- *4 Large russet potatoes*
- *Tablespoon olive oil or vegetable oil*
- *As Needed Traeger Prime Rib Rub*
- *Cup chicken or beef gravy (homemade or jarred)*
- *1 1/2 cup white or yellow cheddar cheese curds*
- *As Needed freshly ground black pepper*
- *2 Tablespoon scallions*

Steps:

1. Set the temperature to maximum when about to cook and preheat, lid shut for 15 minutes.
2. Scrub potatoes into baked, wedge or preferred form and slice them.
3. In a wide mixing bowl, put the potatoes and cover with oil. Cover with Traeger Prime Rib rub generously.

4. Push the potatoes onto a baker's rim and stretch them into a single plate, split down the edges.

5. Roast for 20 minutes and then switch the potatoes to the other side with a spatula. Keep roasting for around 15 to 20 minutes until the potatoes are tender and golden brown.

6. Heat the gravy on your stovetop or in a thermal-proof cup on your Traeger as you roast potatoes.

7. Arrange the potatoes in a wide shallow bowl or on a serving dish to mount the poutine. Distribute the curds of the cheese upwards. Pour over potatoes and cheese curds the hot gravy evenly.

8. Season with black pepper and garnish with slim slices. Serve instantly.

29. SMOKED TROUT DIP

PREP TIME: 2 Hours

COOK TIME: 2 Hours

SERVES: 4 - 6 People

Flaky, brined smoked trout transformed into a creamy and savory dip you won't be able to walk away from.

Ingredients:

- *1 Quart water*
- *1 cup salt*
- *1/2 cup brown sugar*
- *1 Whole lemon zest*
- *4 Whole bay leaves*
- *1 Tablespoon black peppercorn*

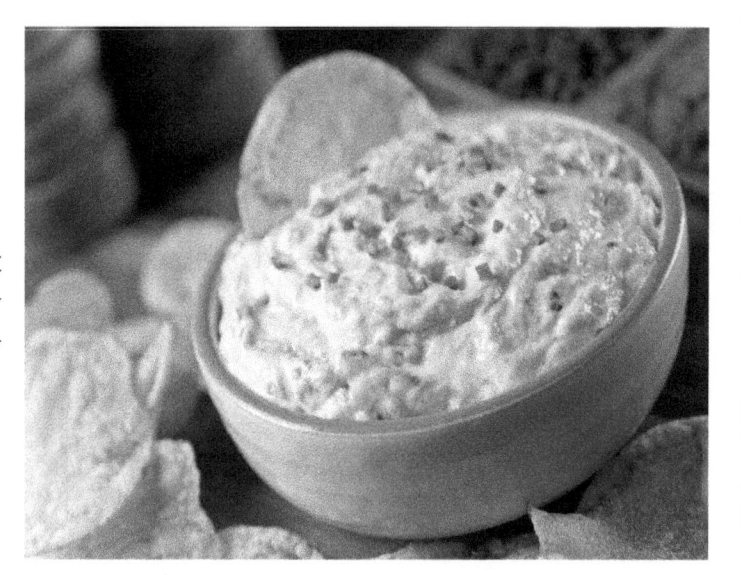

- *2 Pound Trout*
- *1/2 cup cream cheese*
- *1/2 cup sour cream*
- *1 Clove garlic*
- *1/2 Tablespoon parsley, chopped*
- *1/2 Tablespoon chives, chopped*
- *1/2 Tablespoon fresh chopped dill*
- *1 Tablespoon lemon juice*
- *To Taste salt and pepper*

Steps:

1. Layer water, salt, brown sugar, lemon zest, bay leaves and pepper grains in a medium saucepan. Bring to a boil and steam over medium heat until salt and sugar are dissolved. Remove from heat and require 15 minutes to steep. For pouring over ice water to cool. When cold to the touch, combine the trout, cover and chill for 2 hours.

2. Remove the fish from the water. Rinse the fillets. Place them on a cooling rack and cool for the pellicle overnight. This helps the smoke to stick a bit closer to the fillets.

3. Set the temperature to 180°F and preheat for 15 minutes until ready to cook. Set the fillets on the grill directly and smoke for 1-1/2 to 2 hours or until flaking begins.

4. As the trout smokes, combine in a small bowl cream cheese, savory cream, herbs, citrus juice and salt and pepper. Add 1 pound of smooth and smoked trout and mix until the trout breaks into small pieces. Serve with crackers or dip your range of vegetables. Love!

* Cook times differ based on fixed temperatures and the environment.

30. ROASTED SERRANO WINGS

PREP TIME: 1 Day

COOK TIME: 45 Minutes

SERVES: 4 - 6 People

Hot wings are designed to pull the taste buds through the buds. These fire wings are so beautiful, that you can only scream out tears of joy.

Ingredients:

- *4 Pound chicken wings*
- *1 Can beer*
- *2 teaspoon red pepper flakes*
- *As Needed Traeger Cajun Shake*
- *1 Pound serranochile peppers*
- *4 Clove garlic*
- *1 teaspoon Oregano, fresh*
- *1 teaspoon Basil, fresh*
- *1/2 teaspoon Celery Salt*
- *1/4 teaspoon black pepper*
- *1 cup distilled white vinegar*

Steps:

1. In a wide bowl, place the wings and brush them with beer and red pepper flakes. Cool 12–24 hours before grilling.

2. Drop brine wings and pat off. Cut the wings into flats and drummettes. Cut the wing tips — Season liberally throughout with Traeger Chicken Rub.

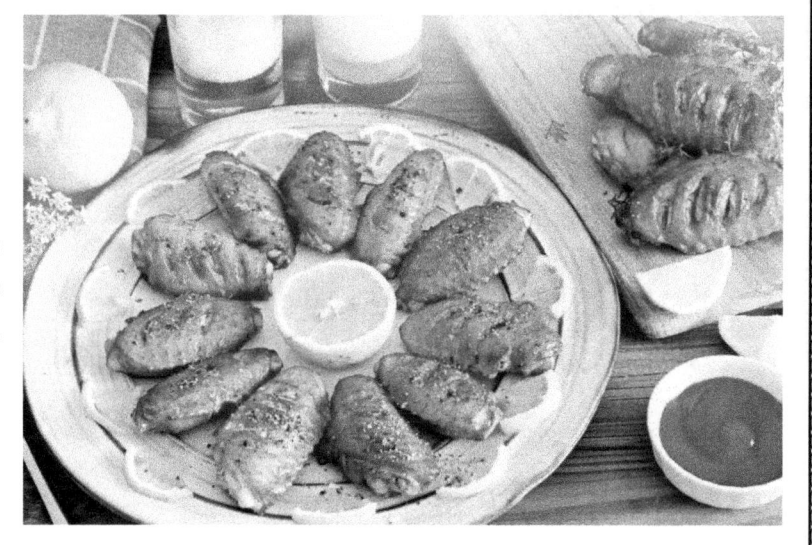

3. Set the traeger at 325°F and preheat it, lid closed for 15 minutes when ready to cook.

4. Place the wings and the peppers on the grill directly. Flip the peppers and barbecue for another 5–10 minutes after 10 minutes or until the skin has roast and hardened. Remove the peppers and the chicken wings off the grill. Allow wings another 20–25 minutes to cook when making the hot sauce.

5. Cut the stems off chili peppers, cut and throw in the garlic, oregano, basil, celery salt and black pepper in a food processor. Turn on the food processor and gently add the vinegar onto the entire mixture.

6. Pour about ½ cup of sauce into a bowl and barbecue; dip the wing in sauce and return to the barbecue for about 5 minutes.

31. WHOLE ROASTED CAULIFLOWER WITH GARLIC PARMESAN BUTTER

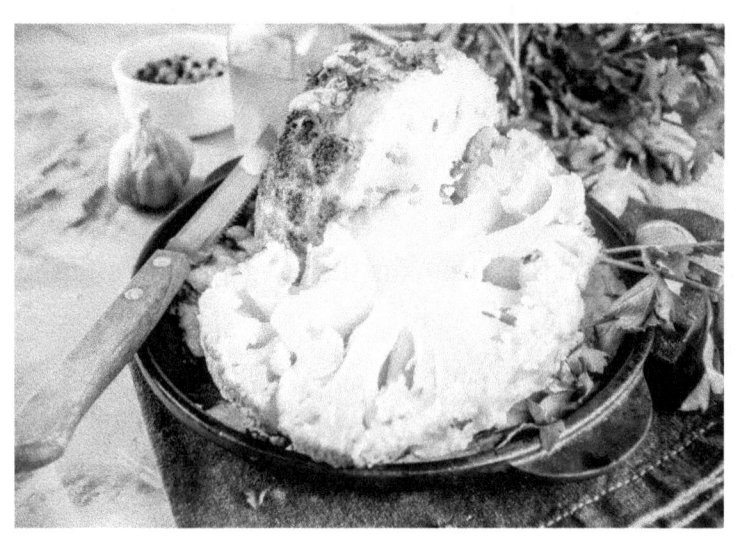

PREP TIME: 15 Minutes

COOK TIME: 45 Minutes

SERVES: 4 - 6 People

Who says cauliflower has to be bland and boring? We bring the flavor with our whole roasted cauliflower. This simple cauliflower recipe will surprise you with how tasty this veggie can be.

Ingredients:

- *1/4 cup olive oil*
- *To Taste salt and pepper*
- *1 Whole Cauliflower, fresh*
- *1/2 cup butter, melted*
- *1/4 cup Parmesan cheese, grated*
- *2 Clove garlic, minced*
- *1/2 Tablespoon parsley, chopped*

Steps:

1. Set the temperature to maximum when about to cook and preheat, lid shut for 15 minutes.
2. Brush with olive oil the cauliflower and season with salt and pepper liberally.

3. Put in a cast iron pan and grill directly and cook for 45 minutes until gold brown and tender core.

4. Combine melted butter, parmesan, garlic and parsley in a small bowl while cooking.

5. In the last 20 minutes of preparation, heat the butter mixture and baste the cauliflower.

6. Remove the cauliflower from the grill and finish with additional parmesan and parsley if needed.

32. SMOKED BEET-PICKLED EGGS

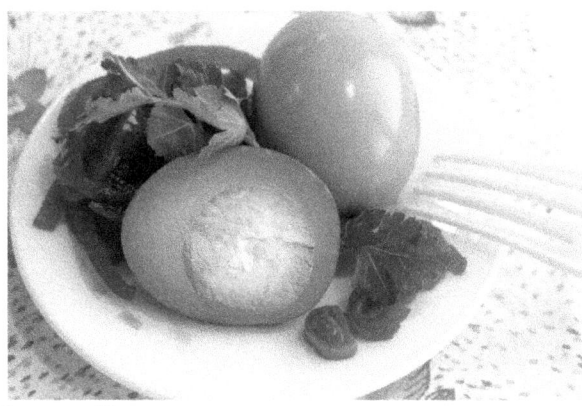

PREP TIME: 30 minutes

COOK TIME: 20 minutes

SERVES: 4-6 people

A show stopper for the Easter table is the bright flavor of beet-pickled shells. This unforgettable appetizer is as tasteful as fun.

Ingredients:

- *6 Eggs, hard-boiled*
- *1 Red Beets, scrubbed and trimmed*
- *1 cup apple cider vinegar*
- *1 cup Beet, juice*
- *1/4 Onion, Sliced*
- *1/3 cup granulated sugar*
- *3 Cardamom*
- *1 star anise*

Steps:

1. Start the Traeger grill and set the temperature to 275°F until ready to cook. Lid locked, preheat for 10 to 15 minutes.

2. Put the hard-boiled peeled eggs on the grill directly and smoke for 30 minutes.

3. Put the smoked eggs in a quarter-size glass jar with the bottom of the cooked/cut beets.

4. Add the vinegar, beet juice, onion, sugar, cardamom and anise in a medium saucepan.

5. Bring to a boil until sugar has dissolved and the onions are translucent (approximately 5 minutes).

6. Remove from heat and leave a few minutes to cool.

7. Pour the combination of vinegar and onions over the eggs and beets in the container, coating completely the eggs.

8. Close the jar firmly. Fun for up to a month.

33. BAKED ARTICHOKE DIP

PREP TIME: 15 Minutes

COOK TIME: 1 Hour

SERVES: 8 - 12 People

Italian Parmesan, Fontina, and Provolone cheeses are combined with smooth and savory dip with artichokes and rusted garlic. Serve with a toasted baguette for the best Traeger appetizer.

Ingredients:

- *10 Clove garlic, peeled*
- *As Needed olive oil*
- *1/2 cup Parmesan cheese*
- *1/2 cup Asiago Cheese*
- *1/2 cup Fontina Cheese*
- *1/2 cup provolone cheese*
- *8 Ounce cream cheese*
- *1/2 cup mayonnaise*
- *1 Can Artichokes*
- *As Needed salt and pepper*

Steps:

1. Set the temperature to 350°F and preheat for 15 minutes until ready to cook. In a tiny oven-safe bowl, place garlic cloves and add enough olive oil to cover the garlic. Cook on the grill for 35–40 minutes. Garlic is done when it is soft enough to quickly push a fork through the garlic. Put away from the barbecue and let it cool.

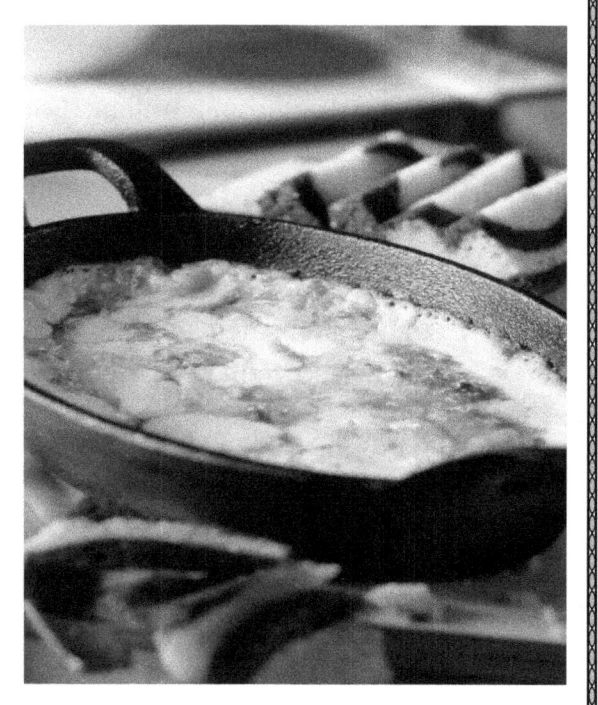

2. Separate the garlic and oil upon cooling and conserve the garlic oil to use in other recipes. In a cup, place the garlic and mash it with a fork until the paste is smooth. Add a bit of garlic-oil if it seems dry.

3. Blend Parmesan, Italian, Fontina and Provolon. Set aside 1/2 cup of mixture of cheeses to finish the sauce.

4. Combine cream cheese, mayonnaise, garlic and artichokes to the cheese mixture. Mix well and add to taste salt and pepper.

5. In an oven-safe pan place mixture and top with 1/2 cup of reserved cheeses. Place the dip at 350°F on the grill and bake for 60 minutes.

6. Eat dip with baguette, cracker, or veggies diced. Serve. Love!

* Cook times differ based on fixed temperatures and the environment.

34. SMOKED SPICY VENISON JERKY

PREP TIME: 20 Minutes

COOK TIME: 5 Hours

SERVES: 6 - 8 People

Take your wild game and turn it into wildly satisfying jerky. Thinly sliced venison marinated in some rich flavor and seasoned with red pepper flakes, cayenne and habanero for some lingering spice.

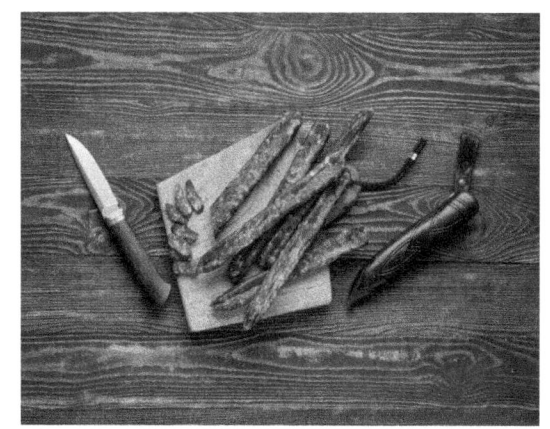

Ingredients:

- *2 Pound venison, trimmed*
- *1 teaspoon apple cider vinegar*
- *1/2 teaspoon onion powder*
- *1 teaspoon granulated garlic*
- *1 teaspoon salt*
- *1/2 cup soy sauce*
- *1/2 cup Worcestershire sauce*
- *1 Tablespoon brown sugar*
- *2 teaspoon black pepper*
- *1 teaspoon paprika*
- *2 teaspoon cayenne pepper*
- *2 teaspoon red pepper flakes*
- *2 habanero peppers, minced*

Steps:

1. Slice the venison into 1/4-inch-thick slices with a sharp knife. Protein or connective tissue is removed.
2. Add all ingredients except venison to a bowl and whisk. Add slices of venison and mix to combine.
3. Transfer bowl contents into a large resealable bag and try to remove the most air. Place in the fridge to marinate overnight.
4. Set Traeger temperature to 180°F when ready to cook and preheat, lid closed for 15 minutes.
5. Remove the venison from the marinade.
6. Arrange the beef directly on the grill in a single plate. Sprinkle with more cayenne powder, red pepper flakes and black pepper for super hot jerky.
7. Smoke for 4 to 5 hours or until the jerky is dry, but chewy and soft when you turn it.
8. Remove from the grill and switch to a cooling rack and cool for 1 hour. Store in the refrigerator in an airtight container or resealable bag.

35. GRILLED BISON SLIDERS

PREP TIME: 15 Minutes

COOK TIME: 10 Minutes

SERVES: 4 - 6 People

If you're crazy for burgers but not cholesterol, you should try these wild game sliders.

Ingredients:

- *1 lb Pound Buffalo, Ground*
- *3 Clove garlic, minced*
- *Tablespoon Worcestershire sauce*
- *1 Teaspoon salt*
- *1 teaspoon black pepper*

Steps:

1. In a mixing bowl, add the meat of buffalo, garlic, Worcestershire sauce, salt, and pepper. Blend with hands.
2. Shape meat into eight tiny patties. Set on a plate and put in the refrigerator.
3. Set the temperature to maximum when about to cook and preheat, lid shut for 15 minutes.
4. Take the patties from the refrigerator and place them on the grill. Flame the patties on each side for 4 minutes and remove from the flame.
5. Put cheese sliced on patties for the last 2 minutes of cooking to melt if you want to add cheese.
6. To toast buns, grill buns for the last minute of cooking.
7. Serve with your of choice sliced onions, pickles, tomatoes, salads and condiments.

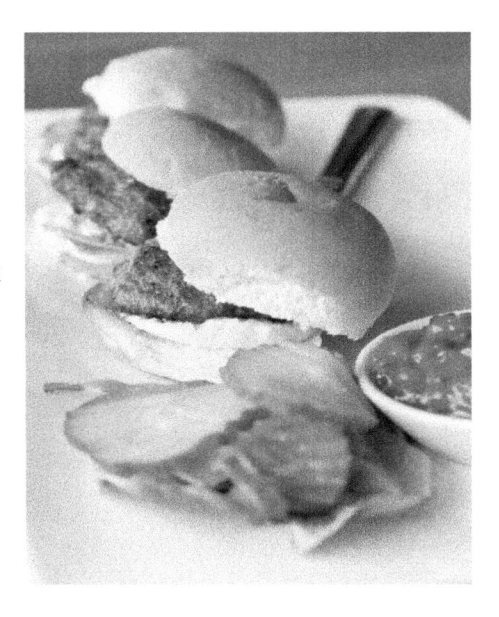

36. BACON WRAPPED CHICKEN WINGS

PREP TIME: 12-24 hours

COOK TIME: 1 hour

SERVES: 2-4 People

If you fire things up with a slice of bacon, wing night will never be the same.

Ingredients:

- *2 Pound chicken wings*
- *24 Ounce beer*
- *2 teaspoon red pepper flakes*
- *To Taste Traeger Cajun Shake*
- *1 Pound bacon*

Steps:

1. Cut the tips off the wings and recycle or hold for the stocks.
2. Cut the skin between the flat and the drummette, leaving the wing a little straighter and simpler to cover.
3. In a wide pot, place the wings and cover with beer and red pepper (if desired). Cool 12–24 hours before grilling.
4. Remove the wings from the brine and clear — season with Cajun Shake Traeger.
5. Wrap each wing in a piece of bacon. If required, you can secure with toothpicks.
6. When ready to cook, start at high temperature (450°F)
7. Directly put the wings on the grill, close the lid, and cook for 30 minutes.
8. Flip the wings and simmer for another 30 minutes or until the chicken is crisp and thoroughly cooked (at least 165°F).

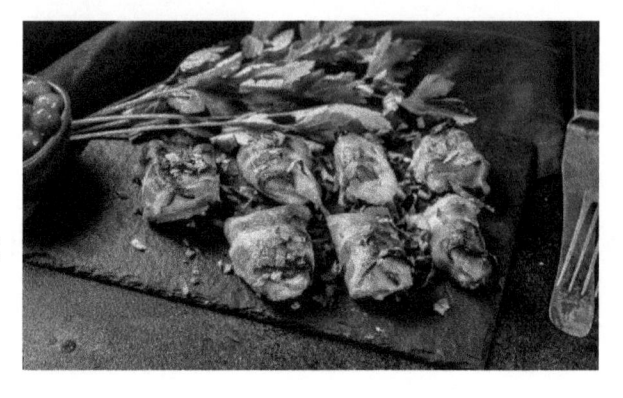

37. PRETZEL ROLLS

PREP TIME: 1 hour,

COOK TIME: 20 minutes,

SERVES: 4-6 persons

You don't have to wait for Oktoberfest for melted pretzel rolls in your mouth, the moist and baked Traegers' bread is wrapped in a fire-grilled brat every year.

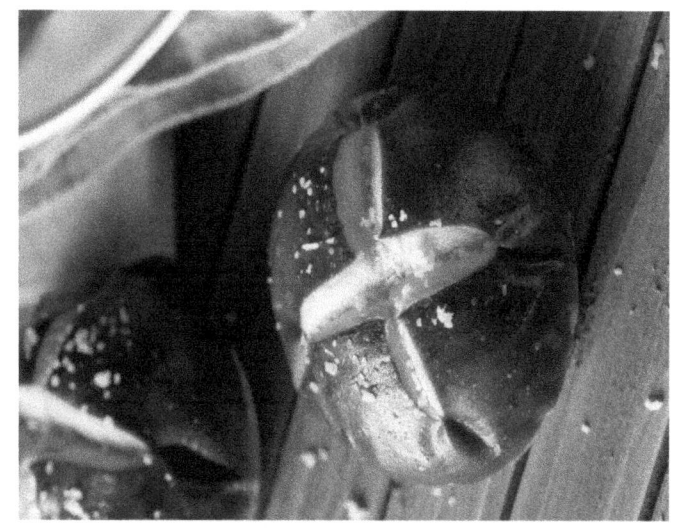

Ingredients:

- *2 3/4 cup Bread Flour*
- *1 Quick-Rising Yeast, envelope*
- *1 teaspoon salt*
- *1 teaspoon sugar*
- *1/2 teaspoon celery seed*
- *1/2 teaspoon Caraway Seeds*
- *1 cup hot water*
- *As Needed Cornmeal*
- *8 cup water*
- *1/4 cup baking soda*
- *2 Tablespoon sugar*
- *1 Whole Egg White*
- *Coarse salt*

Steps:

1. In a food processor or standing blender, mix the bread meal, one envelope yeast, the salt, one tablespoon sugar, the caraway seeds and celery seeds with the dough hook and blend.

2. With the machine going, apply enough water to shape smooth, elastic dough. Knead for 1 minute. (For a few minutes, you could knead it by hand as well.)

3. Small grate bowl. Add the bowl of dough, turning to cover. Cover bowl with plastic wrap, then towel, let the mixture increase in a warm area, about 35 minutes till it doubles in volume.

4. Flour a large baker's sheet. Knead the dough down on a slightly floured surface until smooth. Divide into eight parts. Shape each piece of dough into a disk.

5. Place the balls of dough on the prepared surface, somewhat flattening. Break X into the top of each dough ball by using a sharp knife. Cover with a towel and let the balls of dough rise for 20 minutes.

6. When you are ready to cook, open the Traeger on smoke before a fire has started up (4–5 minutes). Switch 375°F (190°C) temperature and preheat, lid closed, 10 to 15 minutes.

7. Grease another baking sheet and brush with maize meal. Bring water in a large bowl to boil. Add soda and sugar (water sprays). Add three rolls (or many fit comfortably into the pot) and cook 30 seconds on each side.

8. Move rolls to a ready sheet use a slotted knife, place X side up. Do the same with other rolls. Brush rolls with egg white glaze. Generously sprinkle the rolls with coarse salt.

9. Bake rolls around 20 to 25 minutes before dark. Switch to racks and relax 10 minutes. Serve rolls at room temperature or hotter.

38. MINI SAUSAGE ROLLS

PREP TIME: 15 minutes

COOK TIME: 25 minutes

SERVES: 4-6 people.

These sausage pastries are a finger-food breakfast or lunch that can match your soft and tasty palate. We added a honey mustard mix, but feel free to add any of your favorites sauce them.

Ingredients:

- *3/4 cup dry mustard*
- *3/4 cup distilled white vinegar*
- *1/2 cup honey*
- *2 Egg Yolk, Beaten*
- *2 Pound Sausage, Uncooked*
- *To Taste ground sage*
- *1 Small Onion, small diced*
- *17 1/2 Ounce frozen puff pastry*
- *2 Egg Yolk, Beaten*

Steps:

1. Create the mustard: In a mixing pot, add the mustard with the vinegar. Cover with plastic wrap to make sure that the flavors are formulated overnight at room temperature. Transfer to a medium strong saucepan and add sugar and egg yolks to the mustard mixture. Cook on low fire, whisk constantly, about 7 minutes, until thickened. Cool, then chill before it is consumed.

2. Combine the sausage and onion completely in a small mixing bowl. Form each slice of thawed puff pastry—two in a box—on a lightly floured work surface into an 11 by 10-1/2-inch rectangle.

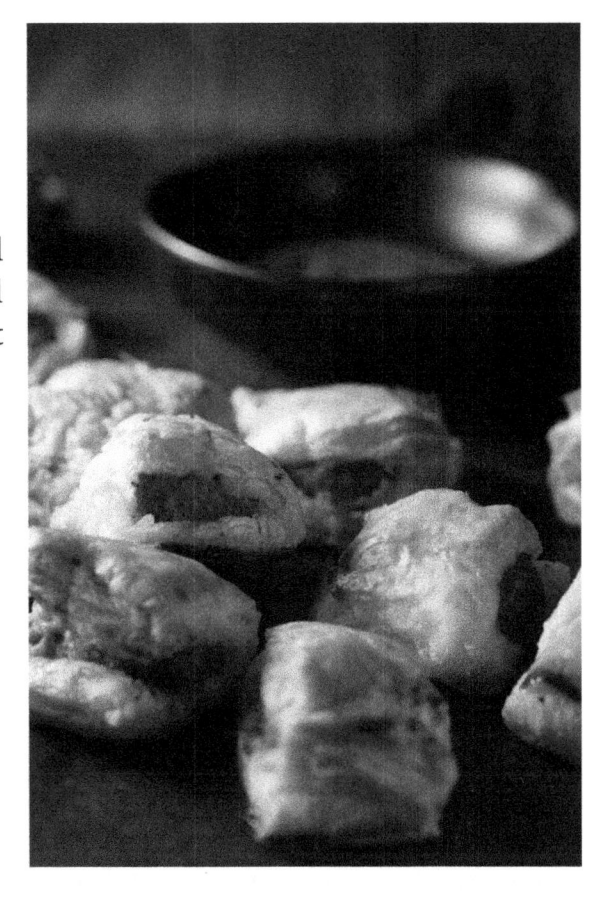

3. Cut each rectangle in width into three strips, each 3-1/2 inch broad, using a pizza cutter or knife. Wet your hands and shape some of your sausages like a funnel. Place it down in the center of one of the bagpipes.

4. Wrap the pastry around the sauce and seal it with a little battered egg. Continue with the sausage and puff pastry left. On the working surface, put all the rolls seam side down and brush the tops gently with the egg.

5. Cut rolls in parts approximately 1-1/2 inches long and move to a rimmed sheet of parchment paper. Leave between each roll about one inch. Set the grill temperature to 350°F and heat it before cooking, lid closed for 15 minutes.

6. Bake the rolls for around 25 minutes or until the sausages are baked and the pastry is golden brown. Serve hot with the mustard sweetheart.

39. ROASTED SWEET POTATO FRIES

PREP TIME: 15 minutes

TIME COOK: 30 minutes

SERVES: 4-6 people

Here we have three Ss: sweet, savory, and spicy. Roast up and let these spuds dive into a chipotle flavor bowl, rendering it the ideal side.

Ingredients:

- *4 Whole sweet potatoes*
- *3 Tablespoons extra-virgin olive oil*
- *1 Tablespoon salt*
- *1 teaspoon black pepper*
- *1 cup mayonnaise*
- *2 Whole Chipotle Peppers in Adobo Sauce*
- *2 Whole lime, juiced*

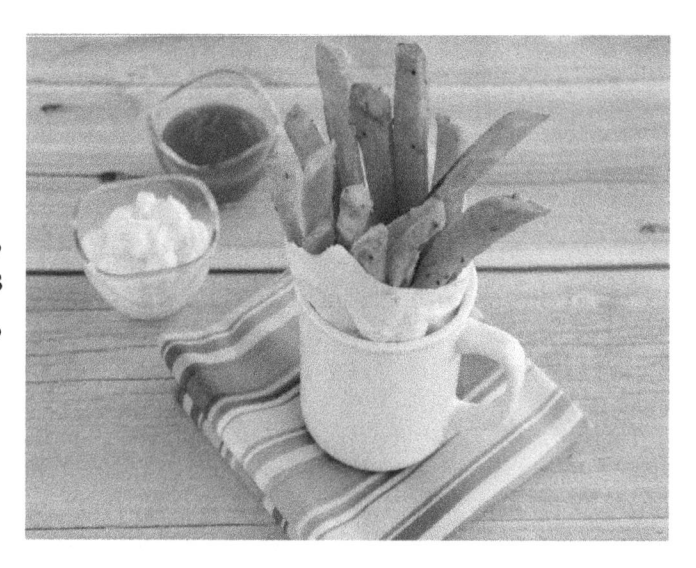

Steps:

1. Set the temperature to maximum when about to cook and preheat, lid shut for 15 minutes.

2. Drop in the olive oil, salt and pepper, the sweet potatoes, and place them on a pan. Place the pan straight on the grill and cook for 20–30 minutes, occasionally stirring until cooked and crispy.

3. Place mayonnaise, chiles and lime juice in a blender and puree until smooth when cooking.

40. BRISKET BURNT END NACHOS

PREP TIME: 20 minutes

COOK TIME: 8 hours

SERVES: 4 to 6 persons

Tender, saucious burnt ends are put with melty cheddar and Monterey Jack cheese on tortilla chips and filled with your preferred toppings.

Ingredients:

- *1 Whole packer brisket*
- *As Needed Traeger Beef Rub*
- *As Needed Traeger 'Que BBQ Sauce*
- *1 Whole Yellow Corn Chips*
- *1 Whole Shredded Mexican Cheese*
- *To Taste Pico De Gallo*
- *To Taste jalapeno, sliced into rings*
- *16 Ounce sour cream*
- *To Taste Guacamole*

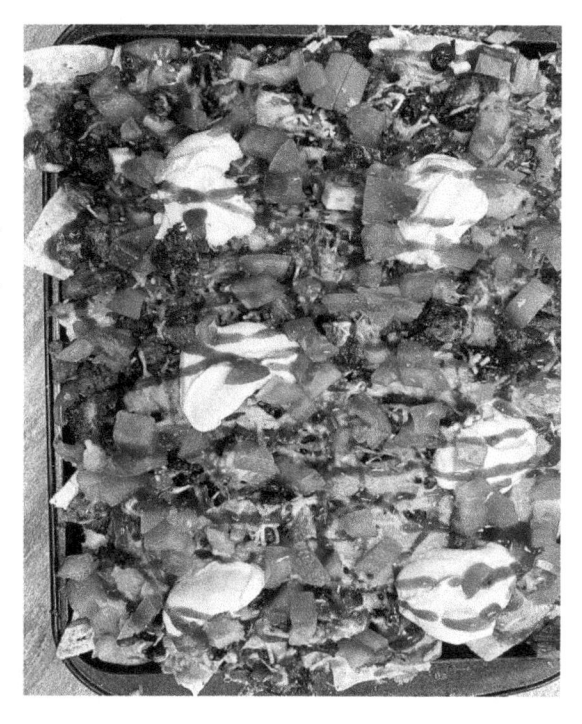

- *1 Bunch Green Onions, Thinly Sliced*
- *1 Bunch cilantro, finely chopped*

Steps:

1. Start the Traeger grill when ready to cook. Set the temperature to 275°F and preheat for 10 to 15 minutes, lid closed.

2. Take off the extra fat and silverskin. Also, remove some "strong" bits of fat so they are not made during cooking. Cut the fat off the bottom of the brisket leaving only 1/4 inch (6 mm) of skin.

3. Two muscles compound a brisket; the point (fat top) and the wide edge (lean top). You ought to butcher the brisket a bit harder than you will with a typical packer in order to prepare brisket burnt ends. Therefore you have to start separating the flat shape of the point after the typical brisket butchering. In short, the fat layer between the point and the flat will be eliminated. Expose the point meat with a sharp knife so that it can consume smoke.

4. Season free with Holy Cow BBQ Rub Meat Church. Put the brisket in your Traeger. If the beef hits an internal temperature of 160°F, double seal the brisket in Traeger paper or aluminum foil using your instant reading thermometer. We name this the Texas crutch. At this stage, the bark would have shaped beautifully.

5. Continue to smoke brisket until the internal temperature exceeds 195°F. The brisket is not completely finished at this time, but the point must be divided to make burnt ends. Remove the brisket and clear the point from the flat. Cover the flat again and give it off to the smoker.

6. Continue to smoke until the meat is "sample tender," which means that there is no resistance when you test it with an instant-read thermometer. Please put a toothpick in a cake and take it out. Every piece of meat is special, but it'll usually be around 203°F at an internal temperature.

7. Rest your brisket for at least an hour in a more refreshing place. Take the point and break into cubes of 1 inch. In the aluminum pan, place the cubes. Season and put more Traeger Beef Rub on the cubes. Fill the cubes with 'Que sauce' from Traeger's. Then vigorously flip the cubes to make sure they are fully filled.

8. Return the pot to the smoker and cook for 1-2 hours, or until the whole liquid has decreased. Enable a few minutes to cool and create nachos.

9. Turn on the Traeger grill according to grill directions when you are ready to cook. Set the temperature to 350°F and preheat for 10 to 15 minutes, lid closed.

10. Place a chip layer, cheese, another chip layer and more cheese. Add the crunchy burnt ends and cook in Traeger for 10 minutes or until the cheese is melted. Top nachos with pico de gallo, green onion, jalapeños, sour cream, guacamole and cilantro.

41. OYSTERS TRAEGEFELLER

PREP TIME: 10 Minutes

COOK TIME: 15 Minutes

SERVES: 2 - 4 People

These are as rich as the New Orleans culture they come from and in the name of Rockefeller, we're bringing you smoky, wood-fired oysters, "Traegefeller." Greens, bacon and cheese to name a few, shell out the ridiculous flavor.

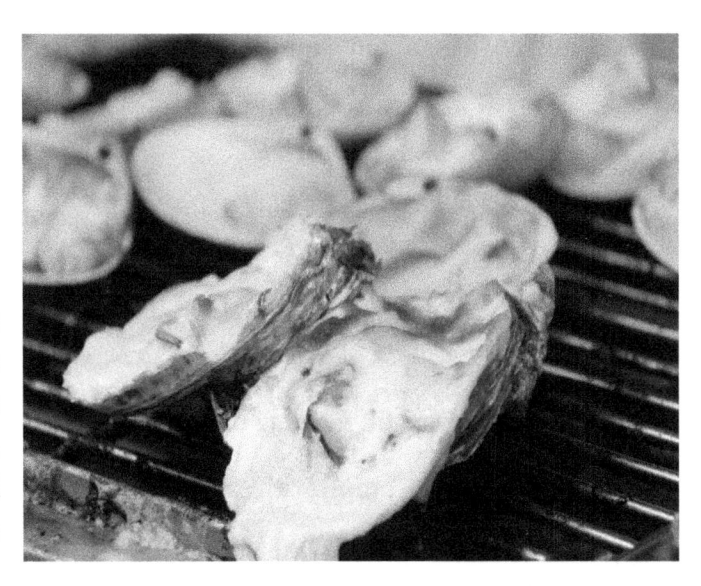

Ingredients:

- *1 Tablespoon butter*
- *1 Shallot, finely chopped*
- *2 cup Collard Greens, fresh*
- *3 Clove garlic, minced*
- *1/4 cup Pernod*
- *1/2 cup Cream*
- *1 cup BBQ chips, crushed*
- *1 cup Parmesan cheese*
- *3 Slices bacon*
- *12 Oysters*

- *As Needed Rock Salt*
- *2 lemon wedges*
- *To Taste salt and pepper*

Steps:

1. In a medium saucepan, melt butter over medium-high flame. Add shallot and collar greens and cook for about 3 minutes until smoothed. Add garlic and sauté until fragrant for 1 minute.

2. Deglaze with Pernod and cook until halved. Add cream and cook 3 minutes, or before the liquid covers a spoon's neck.

3. Combine crushed potato chips, crispy bacon pieces and melted Parmesan cheese in a little bowl.

4. Start the Traeger grill and set the temperature to 500°F until ready to cook. Lid locked, 10 to 15 minutes preheat.

5. Spoon 1 teaspaon heaping on each oyster and a spoonful of the mixture of the potato chips.

6. Sprinkle a pan amply with salt from the block. Place the oysters in the salt to hold them stable.

7. Place on the grill directly and cook 10-15 minutes until golden brown is bubbling. Serve with wedges of lemon.

42. SMOKED TROUT

PREP TIME: 10 Minutes

COOK TIME: 2 Hours

SERVES: 6 - 8 People

This easy smoked trout recipe allows the fish and smoke flavors to shine on their own. Simply butterfly the trout, brine for an hour, let it smoke, then serve it up hot or cold.

Ingredients:

- *8 rainbow trout fillets*
- *1 Gallon water*
- *1/4 cup salt*
- *1/2 cup brown sugar*
- *1 Tablespoon black pepper*
- *2 Tablespoon soy sauce*

Steps:

1. Clean and butterfly fresh food.

2. For brine: Mix one gallon cater, brown sugar, soy sauce, salt and pepper, then mix to absorb salt and sugar. Brine the trout for 60 minutes in the refrigerator.

3. Set Traeger temperature to 225°F when ready to cook and preheat, lid shut for 15 minutes. Using Super Smoke if necessary for optimum taste.

4. Taking the fish out of the brine and pat dry. Place fish directly on barbecue, depending on the thickness of the trout, for 1-1/2 to 2 hours. Fish is finished when it becomes opaque and flakes. Serve warm or cold.

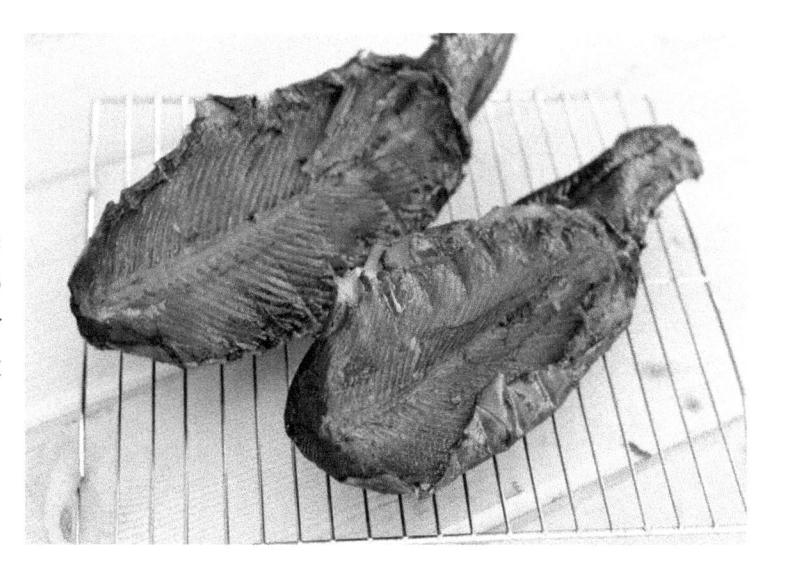

43. TURKEY JALAPEÑO MEATBALLS

PREP TIME: 15 Minutes

COOK TIME: 20 Minutes

SERVES: 8 - 12 People

Our turkey jalapeño meatballs are the perfect mash-up of heat and sweet. Grill them to golden brown on the Traeger & dip them in sweet cranberry glaze.

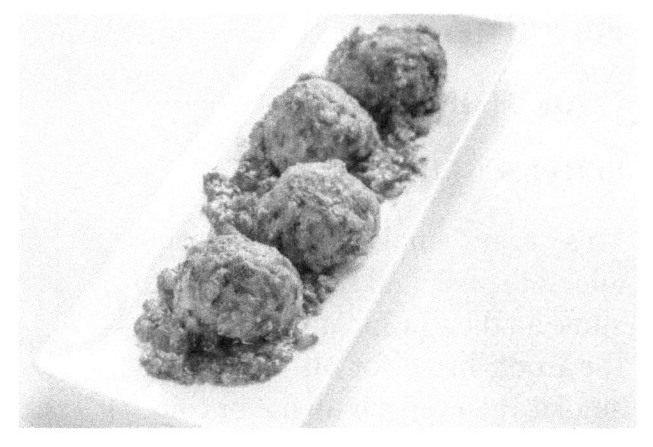

Ingredients:

- *1/4 cup milk*
- *1/2 cup bread crumbs*
- *1 1/4 Pound Turkey, ground*
- *1/2 teaspoon garlic salt*
- *1 teaspoon onion powder*
- *1 teaspoon salt*
- *1/2 teaspoon ground black pepper*
- *1/4 Worcestershire sauce*
- *1 Pinch cayenne pepper*
- *1 Large egg, beaten*
- *1 Whole Jalapeño, seeded and diced*
- *1 cup Cranberry sauce, jellied*
- *1/2 cup Marmalade, Orange*
- *1/2 cup Broth, chicken*
- *To Taste salt and pepper*

Steps:

1. Combine the milk and bread crumbs in a different shallow dish.

2. Mix beef, garlic salt, onion powder, salt, pepper, Worcestershire sauce, egg and jalapeños in a big bowl.

3. Fill in the bowl with the bread crumb milk mixture. Cover with plastic for up to 1 hour and cool.

4. When ready to grill, set the barbecue temperature at 350°F and preheat for 15 minutes.

5. Shape the turkey mixture into balls, around one tablespoon each, and put the meatballs on a parchment-lined baking sheet in a single layer.

6. Cook meatballs until browned and often turn until they exceed 175°F internal temperature and brown all the sides (around 20 minutes).

7. Glaze: In a tiny saucepan, mix cranberry, jelly, chicken broth and jalapeños and steam over medium heat. Cook until ingredients are combined.

8. Brush the meatballs with the cranberry glaze halfway into the meatball cook.

9. Move meatballs to serving plates with cranberry glaze. Serve instantly.

44. BACON WRAPPED CHERRY TOMATOES

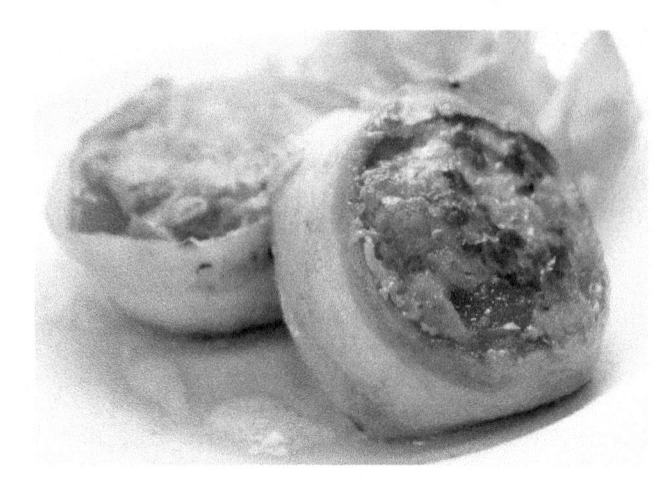

PREP TIME: 15 Minutes

COOK TIME: 25 Minutes

SERVES: 4 - 6 People

This bite-sized appetizer is perfect for sharing. Serve with balsamic vinegar for dipping at your next get-together.

Ingredients:

- *20 Tomatoes, cherry*
- *10 Slices bacon*
- *As Needed Toothpicks, wooden*
- *To Taste cracked black pepper*
- *To Taste balsamic vinegar*
- *To Taste Basil, fresh*

Steps:

1. Turn on the Traeger and load it to 500°F. Lid locked, preheat 10 to 15 minutes.
2. Slice the bacon part way back. Wrap each tomato half a slice of bacon in a wooden toothpick and lock it.
3. Put tomatoes on a large sheet of foil and sprinkle with cracked black pepper.
4. Cook the tomatoes on the Traeger for about 25 minutes or until the bacon has been made and the tomatoes burst.
5. Remove tomatoes and serve warm with fresh basil and a drizzle of balsamic vinegar, if desired.

45. GRILLED BLOOMING ONION

PREP TIME: 15 Minutes

COOK TIME: 30 Minutes

SERVES: 4 - 6 People

No need to go to a lousy chain steak house anymore for a blooming onion, you can now make this iconic dish right in your backyard with minimal effort.

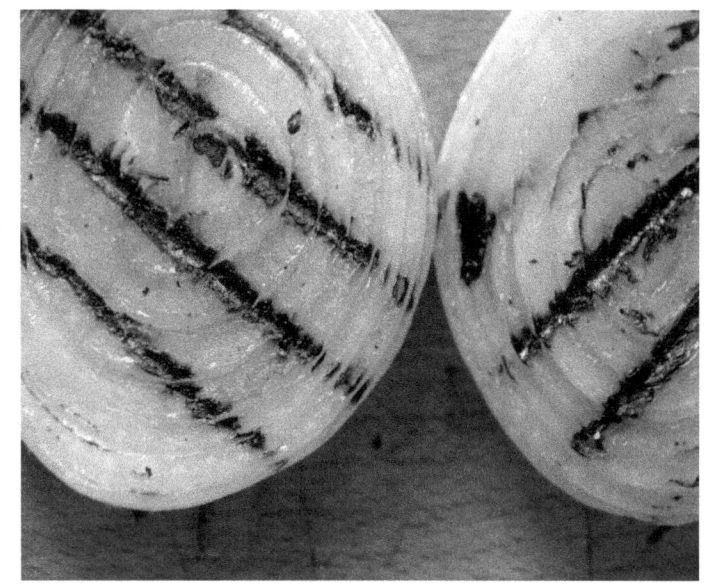

Ingredients:

- *1 Large Vidalia Onion*
- *4 cups all-purpose flour*
- *1/4 cup granulated garlic*
- *1/4 cup onion powder*
- *4 Tablespoons kosher salt*
- *1 Tablespoon black pepper*
- *1 Tablespoon paprika*
- *2 Tablespoons cayenne pepper*
- *1/2 Tablespoon ground mustard*
- *1 Tablespoon canola oil*
- *1 Quart buttermilk*
- *To Taste salt and pepper*
- *4 Tablespoons Parmesan Cheese, Shredded*
- *1 Tablespoon fresh parsley*

Steps:

1. Peel the onion, just don't break it off. Cut about 1/2" from the foundation into eight wedges, make sure you don't carve it all open. Separate the onion pieces carefully.

2. In a medium bowl, combine all ingredients for the coating and mix well. Break the coating in half for two medium bowls.

3. In a small bowl, add buttermilk, season with salt and pepper.

4. In the flour mixture dredge onion, then in buttermilk, and then back in the flour mixture.

5. Place the root side of the onion down onto a sheet of paper-lined sheet and sprinkle with an oil spray.

6. Set the temperature to high and preheat for 15 minutes when ready to cook. In the center of the grill put the tray and cook for 30 minutes.

7. When the onion is cooked and opened, sprinkle the cheese uniformly over the onion and grill for another 2 minutes or until the cheese has melted.

8. Add fresh parsley to the garnish. Serve immediately with your favorite sauces and lemon wedges. Love!

* Cook times differ based on fixed temperatures and the environment.

46. EVERYTHING PIGS IN A BLANKET

PREP TIME: 20 Minutes

COOK TIME: 15 Minutes

SERVES: 4 - 6 People

The hogs on the offensive line will be protecting these pigs in a blanket, a favorite of Todd Fritz from The Dan Patrick Show. When you need a quick and easy appetizer, start the grill and roll these Lil' smokies into their dough uniform.

Ingredients:

- *2 Tablespoons Poppy Seeds*
- *1 Tablespoon Dried Minced Onion*
- *2 teaspoons garlic, minced*
- *2 Tablespoons Sesame Seeds*
- *1 teaspoon salt*
- *8 Ounces Original Crescent Dough*
- *1/4 cup Dijon mustard*
- *1 Large egg, beaten*

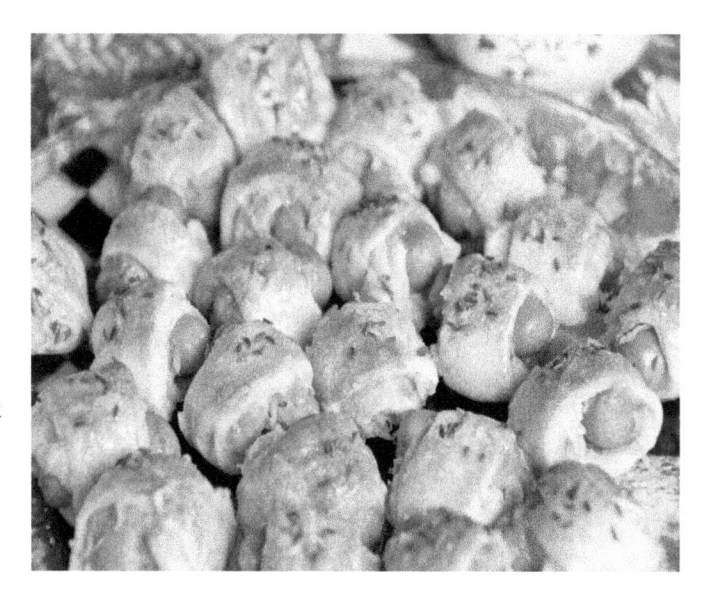

Steps:

1. When you are ready to cook, start your Traeger at 350°F and preheat for 10–15 minutes with the lid closed.
2. Mix the seeds of poppy, dried minced onion, dried minced garlic, salt and sésame. Set aside.
3. Cut each triangle of crescent roll dough into thirds alongside it and make from each roll three small strips.
4. Brush the dough with Dijon mustard gently. Place the hot dogs on the dough end and flip over.
5. Arrange on a greased baking pan, seam side down. Wash with egg and sprinkle with the mixture of seasoning.
6. Bake in Traeger for about 12 to 15 minutes until golden brown.
7. Serve with your choice of mustard or dipping sauce.

47. SPICY CRAB POPPERS

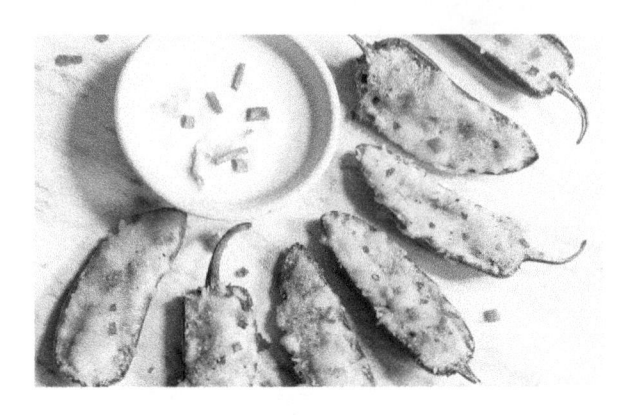

PREP TIME: 20 Minutes

COOK TIME: 30 Minutes

SERVES: 8 - 12 People

This delicious jalapeño poppers recipe will impress every last game-day guest. It's a simple appetizer that's packed with buttery fresh crab & has a bit of kick.

Ingredients:

- *18 Whole jalapeño*
- *8 Ounce cream cheese softened*
- *1 cup Canned Corn, drained*
- *1/2 cup Crab meat, lump*
- *1 1/4 teaspoon Old Bay Seasoning*
- *2 Scallions, minced*

Steps:

1. Cut each jalapeño half-long and cut the ribs and seeds.
2. Combine cream cheese, corn, crab meat, scallions, and Old Bay Seasoning in a mixing pot, and combine until blended. Stir in the scallions. Spoon the jalapeño halves and gently mound it.
3. Arrange the poppers on a foil or parchment-covered baking dish.
4. Once you are ready to cook, start the Traeger grill on Smoke and open the deck before it is set (4 to 5 minutes). Set the temperature to 350°F and preheat for 10 to 15 minutes, lid closed.
5. Roast the jalapeños for 25 to 30 minutes or until the peppers soften and the filling is warm and smooth.
6. Until eating, cool slightly.

48. THAI CHICKEN SKEWERS

PREP TIME: 30 Minutes

COOK TIME: 10 Minutes

SERVES: 4 - 6 People

Take your chicken to new heights. This recipe will take your food and your family's taste buds on a trip to the Far East with flavors such as coconut, ginger, red curry, and cumin.

Ingredients:

- *2 Pound boneless, skinless chicken breast*
- *1 cup cilantro leaves*
- *1/2 cup Coconut Milk, unsweetened*
- *3 Tablespoon lime juice*
- *2 Clove garlic, chopped*
- *1 Small 1" Piece of Ginger, peeled and coarsely chopped*
- *2 Tablespoon brown sugar*
- *1 Tablespoon Thai Red Curry Paste*
- *1 teaspoon cumin*
- *1 teaspoon black pepper*
- *As Needed Peanut Sauce*

Steps:

1. Slice the chicken into 1/2-inch wide strips throughout the line (it is better if the chicken is partially frozen first). Put the strips in a re-selling plastic bag.

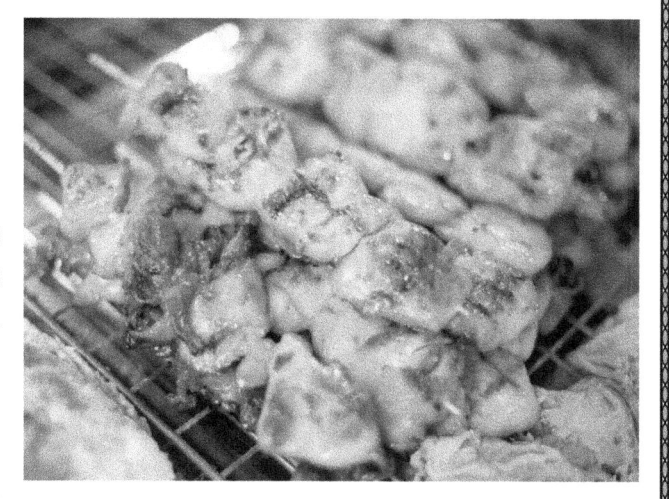

2. Combine the cilantro, coconut milk, lime juice, garlic, ginger, brown sugar, curry paste, cumin and pepper in a mixing container and blend until smooth. Pour over the chicken strips and cool for a minimum of 1 hour.

3. Drain the chicken and throw the marinade away. Insert the chicken strips onto the skewers of bamboo. Start the Traeger grill and set the temperature to 400°F when ready to cook and preheat, covered, for 10 to 15 minutes.

4. Arrange the skewers directly on the grill in two rows. Glide an aluminum foil fragment under the uncovered ends of the skewers to stop them from burning. Grill the chicken until it has been cooked and turn 4 to 5 minutes per side.

5. Serve promptly with peanut sauce.

49. PROSCIUTTO WRAPPED GRILLED SHRIMP WITH PEACH SALSA

PREP TIME: 20 Minutes

COOK TIME: 12 Minutes

SERVES: 4 - 6 People

Your new go-to appetizer. Shrimp is already delicious, but wrap it in prosciutto and serve with peach salsa for an amplified flavor.

Ingredients:

- *2 Pound Shrimp, Peeled & Deveined*
- *8 Slices Prosciutto Ham*
- *Toothpicks*
- *2 Whole Peaches, Diced*
- *2 Tablespoon balsamic vinegar*
- *2 Tablespoons honey*

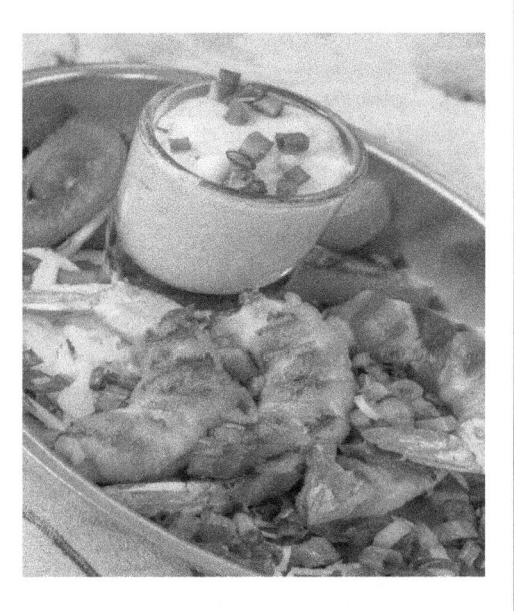

- *1 Chile, serrano chopped*
- *2 Tablespoon Basil, Fresh, Chopped*
- *To Taste salt*
- *To Taste black pepper*

Steps:

1. Rinse the shrimp under cold running water and dry thoroughly on paper towels. Spiral around a slice of prosciutto, secure with a toothpick if you like.
2. Salsa peach: Mix in a pot the peaches, 1 tbsp vinegar, honey, 1/2 serrano pepper, basil, salt and pepper. Apply additional sugar, honey, garlic, salt and pepper to compare.
3. Set the temperature to maximum when about to cook and preheat, lid shut for 15 minutes.
4. Place the shrimp on the grill and barbecue for 4 to 6 minutes, or until shrimp is opaque.
5. Serve the warm shrimp with the fishing salsa. Garnish with jalapenos slices for additional flavor.

50. SMOKED HUMMUS WITH ROASTED VEGETABLES

PREP TIME: 15 Minutes

COOK TIME: 40 Minutes

SERVES: 4 - 6 People

Give this healthy snack some smokin' flavor. This homemade hummus is seasoned with aromatic spices like tahini, garlic, and smoked paprika, smoked, and served aside roasted veggies for the perfect dip.

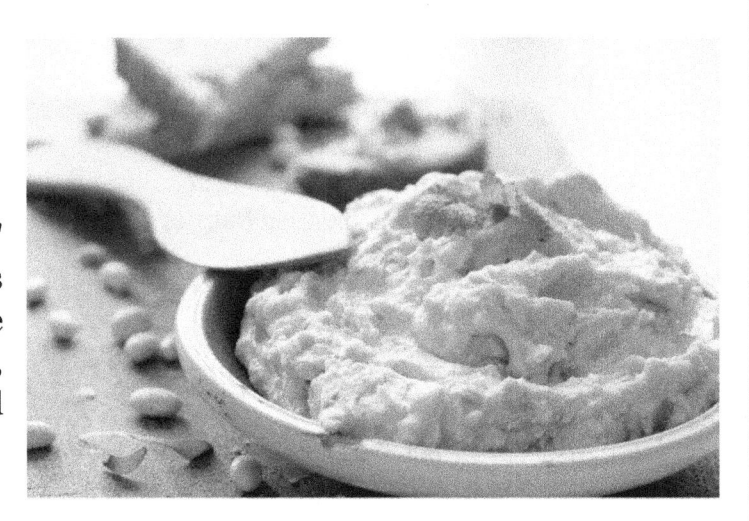

Ingredients:

- *1 1/2 cup Chickpeas*
- *333/1000 cup Tahini*
- *1 Tablespoon garlic, minced*
- *2 Tablespoons extra-virgin olive oil*
- *1 teaspoon salt*
- *4 Tablespoons lemon juice*
- *1 Red Onion, Sliced*
- *2 cups butternut squash*
- *2 cups Cauliflower, cut into florets*
- *2 cups Brussels Sprouts, fresh*
- *2 Whole Portobello Mushroom*
- *4 Tablespoons extra-virgin olive oil*
- *To Taste salt*
- *To Taste black pepper*

Steps:

1. Set the grill temperature to 180°F when ready to cook and preheat, lid closed for 15 minutes.
2. For hummus: drain and rinse chickpeas on a sheet tray, place the casserole in the grill for 15-20 minutes, or smoke to the desired level.
3. Combine chickpeas, tahini, garlic, olive oil, salt and lemon juice in the food processor's bowl and cycle to a fully blended but not absolutely smooth mixture. Take to a cup and set aside.
4. Increase the grill temperature to high and preheat.
5. For vegetables: Drizzle veggies and spray them with olive oil. Place the sheet tray in the grill and roast the vegetables for 15 to 20 minutes before they are gently browned.
6. In a serving bowl or plate, put hummus and cover with roasted veggies.
7. Serve with olive oil and pita bread.

51. GRILLED KOREAN SHORT RIBS

PREP TIME: 8 Hours

COOK TIME: 10 Minutes

SERVES: 4 - 6 People

A homemade Korean marinade and applewood smoke take this wood-fired twist on beef short ribs to the top. These marinated short ribs are sure to be wood-fired showstoppers.

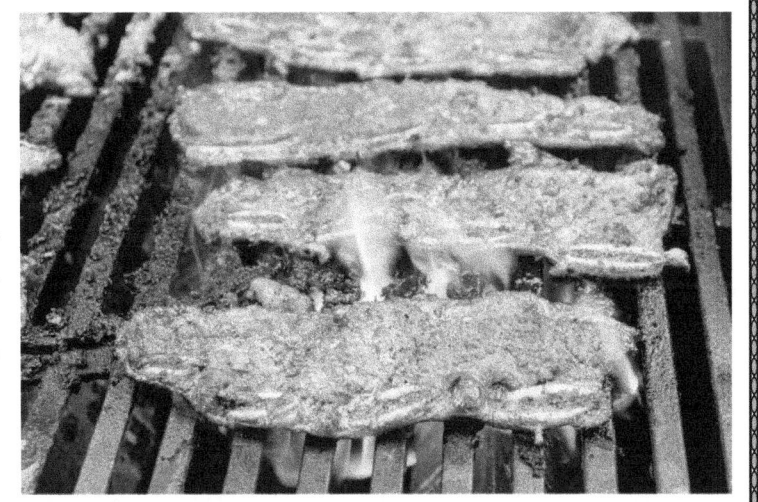

Ingredients:

- *1/2 cup soy sauce*
- *1 cup brown sugar*
- *1/2 cup rice wine vinegar*
- *1 Tablespoon sesame oil*
- *2 Clove garlic*
- *1 Whole 1" Piece of Ginger, peeled and coarsely chopped*
- *1 Whole Asian Pear, peeled and quartered*
- *1 Whole Red Thai Chili, deseeded and chopped*
- *5 Pound Korean Short Ribs*
- *As Needed Sesame Seeds*
- *As Needed Scallions, sliced*

Steps:

1. To produce the marinade, all ingredients are mixed until smooth except for the ribs and puree in the pitcher of a blender. Pour over short ribs, seal and marinate overnight in the refrigerator.

2. Set the temperature to maximum when about to cook and preheat, lid shut for 15 minutes. Set to 500°F if necessary for better performance.

3. Remove marinade ribs and put marinade away. Put the ribs on the grill directly and cook for 3–5 minutes.

4. Take from the grill and add thin scallions or sesame seeds.

52. BBQ CHICKEN DRUMSTICKS

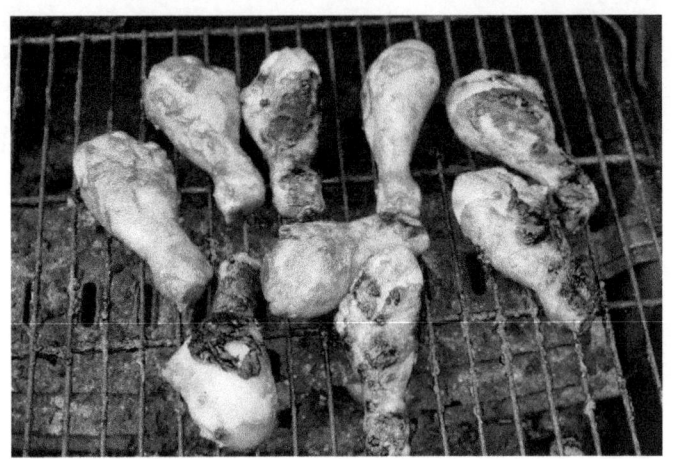

PREP TIME: 15 Minutes

COOK TIME: 2 Hours

SERVES: 4 - 6 People

Celebrate touchdowns and trick-plays with these Traeger drumsticks. Smoked and saucy, Seton O'Connor from The Dan Patrick Show knows this barbecue meat treat is ready for game day action.

Ingredients:

- *8 chicken drumsticks*
- *2 Tablespoon Traeger Chicken Rub*
- *1/2 cup Traeger 'Que BBQ Sauce*

Steps:

1. Season each drumstick and allow 20 minutes to rest.

2. Set the traeger temperature to 275°F and preheat, lid closed for 15 minutes when ready to cook.

3. Hang the drumsticks on the hanger (alternatively, place grate straight on the grill halfway through) and cook 1 hour.

4. Take the drumsticks from the hanger and placed in a bowl.

5. Cover with foil and cook 45 minutes longer or until the inside temperature of meat reaches 190°F.

6. Remove the foil and cover all pan drumsticks with sauce.

7. Heat the sauce for an extra 15 minutes.

8. Remove from Traeger and let stand until served for 15 minutes.

53. SMOKED MUSTARD WINGS

PREP TIME: 10 Minutes

COOK TIME: 55 Minutes

SERVES: 6 - 8 People

Sweet, smoky wings with a tangy mustard kick. These wings are tossed in a warm mustard sauce, grilled, and then smoked for some deep wood-fired flavor.

Ingredients:

- *1/2 cup spicy brown mustard*
- *1 cup apple cider vinegar*
- *1/2 cup soy sauce*
- *2 Tablespoon honey*
- *1 Tablespoon Miso*
- *1/2 cup molasses*
- *5 Pound chicken wings*
- *1/4 cup canola oil*
- *To Taste salt and pepper*
- *As Needed lemon wedges*

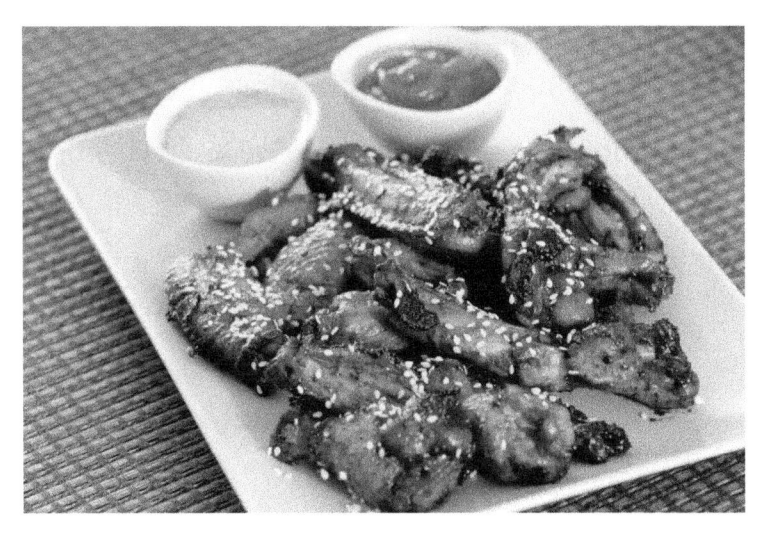

Steps:

1. Whisk the mustard with sugar, molasses, soy sauce, honey and miso in a small saucepan. Carry to simmer. Cook for around 15 minutes over medium heat, stirring regularly until thickened and reduced to 1 cup.

2. Start the Traeger grill and set the temperature at 500°F until ready to cook. Lid locked, preheat 10 to 15 minutes.

3. Throw the chicken wings in a large bowl with the oil and season with salt and pepper.

4. Put the wings on the fire and cook until slightly browned and baked, around 15 minutes. Switch sometimes, so wings don't burn.

5. Reduce the grill temperature to 225°F (and, if available, trigger Super Smoke). For a good 30 minutes, smoke wings.

6. Move the wings to a wide clean bowl with tongs. Mix the wings with the sauce and return to the grill.

7. Increase the temperature to 350°F and start frying, about 10 to 15 minutes longer before glazed and slightly charred in spots.

8. Switch the wings to a plate and decorate with chopped herbs. Serve with wedges of lemon.

54. BEEF SATAY

PREP TIME: 10 Minutes

COOK TIME: 10 Minutes

SERVES: 6 - 8 People

Traeger marinade and garlic invigorate beef with colorful seasonings, and the severe flavor will have your crowd begging for seconds.

Ingredients:

- *2 Pound Black Flat Iron Steak*
- *1 Bottle Carne Asada Marinade, of Choice*
- *2 Clove garlic, minced*
- *2 scallions, chopped*
- *As Needed Peanut Sauce*
- *1/4 cup Peanuts, Crushed*
- *2 Limes*

Steps:

1. Break the steak into 1/3-inch slices on a straight diagonal way with a sharp knife. (Not only does it maximize the strip length, but it also ensures tenderness to the meat) Put into a resealable plastic bag or a large bowl. Pour the marinade of Carne Asada over the beef and apply the scallions and garlic. Cool for 1 hour.

2. Take the beef out of the marinade and pick off any garlic or onion bits. Thread every bit on a skewer of bamboo.

3. Place the Traeger to high and preheat until ready to start, lid closed for 15 minutes.

4. Grill the satays once, 3 to 4 minutes on each hand.

5. Place the peanut sauce in a tiny bowl and place it on one end of a plate or tray. Arrange on the tray the satays and scatter with the peanuts. Garnish with wedges of lime.

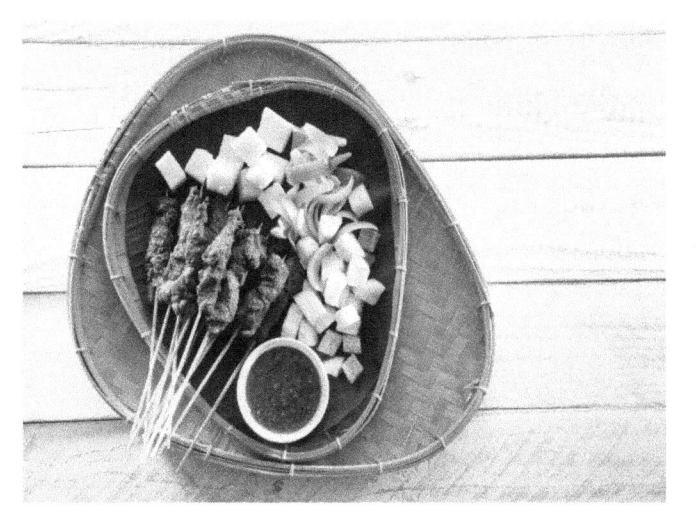

55. BAKED SWEET POTATOES

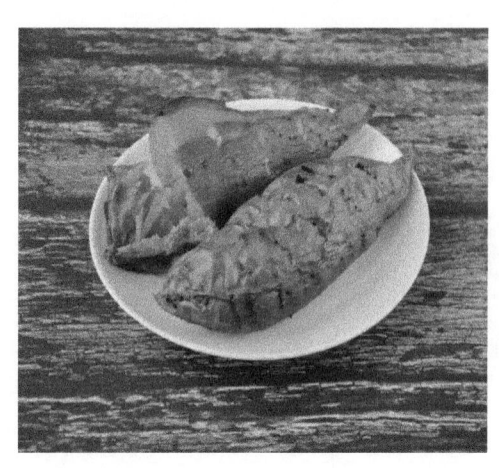

PREP TIME: 15 Minutes

COOK TIME: 1 Hour

SERVES: 8 - 12 People

Wish your sweet potato had more sugared goodness? This recipe was made for the elf you. Maple syrup and cinnamon make this side dish the star of the show. Ask your buddies what the difference between a sweet potato and yam is, then let them yammer on about it.

Ingredients:

- *1 cup butter, softened*
- *1/4 cup pure maple syrup*
- *1/2 teaspoon ground cinnamon*
- *8 Medium sweet potatoes*

Steps:

1. Mix together the butter, maple syrup, cinnamon and whip with a bamboo spoon into a mixing bowl. Move to a small pot, cover and chill before serving time. (Alternatively, combine the ingredients with a hand-hold mixer or a stand blender)

2. When ready to cook, put the sweet potatoes on the Grill and cook for 1-1/2 hours, depending on the size of the potatoes, until tender. Make a cut on either side, then gently pinch the ends to fluff.

3. Serve soft with the butter of Maple-Cinnamon.

56. BAKED LOADED TATER TOTS

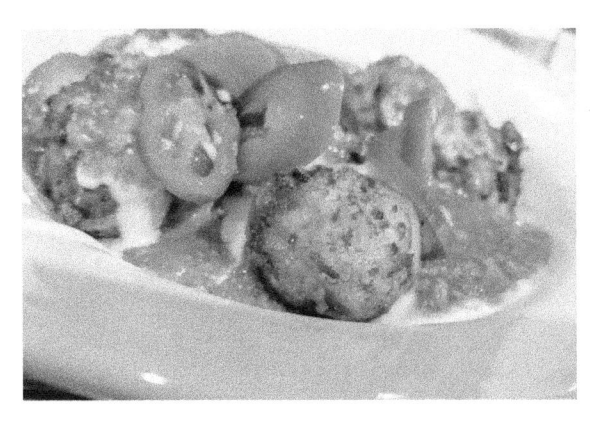

PREP TIME: 10 Minutes

COOK TIME: 35 Minutes

SERVES: 6 - 8 People

You've never seen tots like these before. Loaded with chili, cheesy cheese, onions, and a sour cream drizzle, this is one classic appetizer you'll keep coming back to.

Ingredients:

- *2 Pound Tater Tots, Frozen*
- *1 Can Black Beans*
- *1 1/2 cup leftover chili*
- *1 cup Cheese, Leftover*
- *1 Red Onion, finely diced*
- *1/2 cup cilantro, chopped*
- *1/2 cup sour cream*

Steps:

1. Set the temperature to 375°F and preheat until ready to prepare, lid closed for 15 minutes.
2. Put frozen tots on a plate tray and position on the grill directly.
3. Cook until tots are crispy for 20–25 minutes.
4. Heat chili, cheese and beans. Place on the barbecue for 15 minutes.
5. Remove from the grill and top with red onions, cilantro, sour cream and jalapeno. Love!

57. OLD FASHIONED CORNBREAD

PREP TIME: 10 Minutes

COOK TIME: 25 Minutes

SERVES: 4 - 6 People

This simple cornbread recipe bakes up perfectly in our cornbread skillet. It's infused with delicious smoke flavor and finished with a smear of smoked butter.

Ingredients:

- *1 cup all-purpose flour*
- *1 cup Cornmeal*
- *1 Tablespoon sugar*
- *2 teaspoon baking powder*
- *1/2 teaspoon salt*
- *3 Tablespoon butter*
- *1 cup milk*
- *1 Whole egg, lightly beaten*

Steps:

1. Combine flour, cornmeal, sugar, baking powder and salt in a mixing pot.
2. In a tiny cup, heat the butter. Clear from heat and add milk and egg. (Make sure that the mixture is not soft, or that the egg is curdling.)
3. Add the combination of milk and egg to the dry ingredients and blend together. Do not overmix.
4. Disperse the batter equally into a greased 8 or 9-inch skillet.
5. Start the Traeger grill ready for cooking and set the temperature to 375°F and preheat.
6. Bake the bread until it begins to fall off the sides of the pan and the surface starts to shine, for 25 to 35 minutes. To serve, cut into squares (or wedges, if you used a pastry plate)

58. JALAPEÑO CANDIED SMOKED SALMON

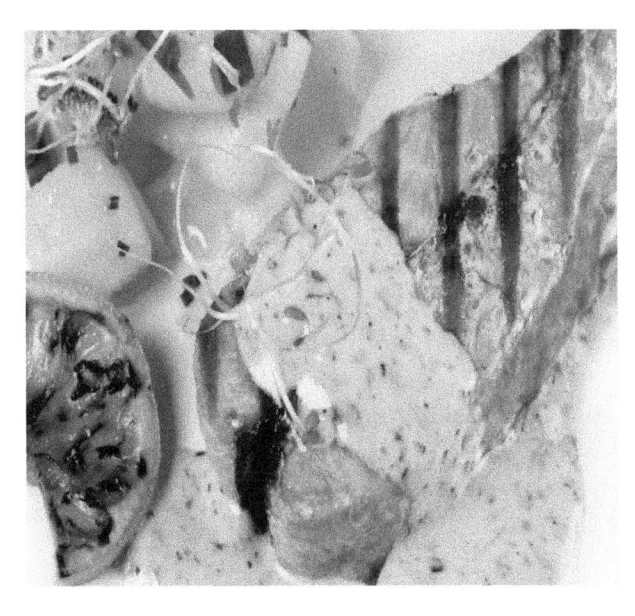

PREP TIME: 4 Hours

COOK TIME: 1 Hour

SERVES: 4 - 6 People

Spicy candied salmon is a delicious snack that's high in protein & easy to take on hikes, a bike ride, or a day on the lake.

Ingredients:

- *1/2 cup hot water*
- *2 whole Jalapeno, chopped*
- *1 To Taste red pepper flakes*
- *1/4 cup soy sauce*
- *1/4 cup sugar*
- *2 Tablespoons garlic powder*
- *2 Tablespoons ground black pepper*
- *8 cups Water, cold*
- *1 Whole Salmon Fillet, pin bones removed*
- *1 cup brown sugar*
- *2 Whole jalapeño*
- *3 Tablespoons Dijon mustard*

Steps:

1. Brine: Mix boiling water, jalapeños and red pepper flakes into a small saucepan. Apply jalapeños and flakes of red pepper to required flame.

2. Bring water to a boil for 5 minutes and steep jalapeños in boiling water. Add the remaining brine ingredients except the cold water and blend before sugar is dissolved.

3. Bringing the cool water into it. After the brine is no longer hot, place the salmon in a wide resealable jar.

4. Cool the salmon in the brine for 3 to 4 hours, depending on the fillet size.

5. Remove salmon from the brine when ready to grill, clean and pat dry.

6. Glaze: In a blender mix brown sugar, jalapeños and Dijon mustard and pump before jalapeños are completely combined. Fill the salmon with the glaze.

7. Set the Traeger to 180°F and preheat, lid closed for 15 minutes before ready to cook.

8. Smoke salmon for 30 minutes on the skin side down.

9. rise rise to 225°F. Steam salmon for 45 minutes up to 1 hour.

10. Remove and drink from the barbecue.

59. GRILLED CORN SALSA

PREP TIME: 25 Minutes

COOK TIME: 15 Minutes

SERVES: 6 - 8 People

Customize this substantial, satisfying salsa recipe to your desired spice level—from a whisper of heat to the blazing inferno. Treat your taste buds to spice balanced by the sweetness of wood-fired corn—your mouth will thank you.

Ingredients:

- *4 Large Corn Husks*
- *4 Tomato, chopped*
- *1/2 cup cilantro, finely chopped*
- *1 red onion, diced*
- *1 teaspoon garlic powder*
- *1 teaspoon onion powder*
- *1 Jalapeno, Grilled, Seeded, and Diced*
- *1 lime, juiced*
- *To Taste salt*

Steps:

1. Set the Traeger to high and preheat until ready to cook, lid closed for 15 minutes.
2. Put the maize on the barbecue and cook until completely charred, scrape the husk and cut the cob's kernels.
3. Combine the maize with the other ingredients and cool before ready to eat. Serve with chips or as an accompaniment to your preference of fiesta dishes.

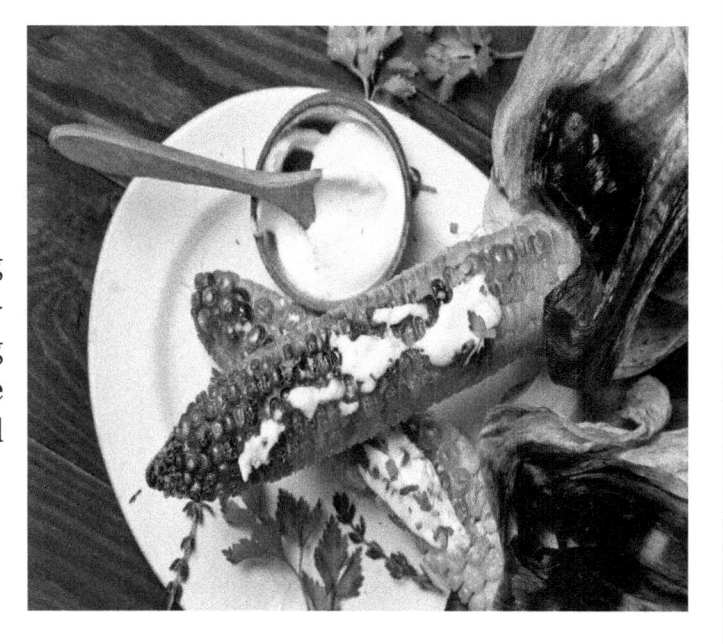

60. TRAEGER MANDARIN WINGS

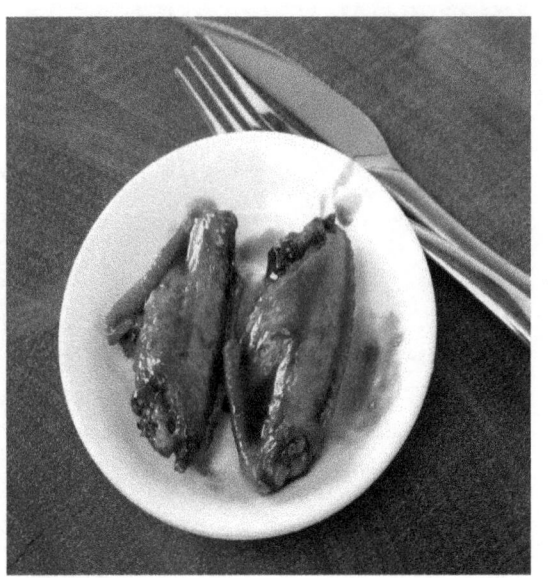

PREP TIME: 5 Minutes

COOK TIME: 30 Minutes

SERVES: 2 - 4 People

It's getting a little sweet but a lot of spicy up in here. Whether your wings are dripping in glaze or dry, shower them with savory Traeger Rubs and grill. It's wing night at your house, and there's nothin' mild about it.

Ingredients:

- *1 Bottle Mandarin glaze*
- *As Needed Traeger Beef Rub*
- *As Needed Traeger Chicken Rub*
- *2 Pound chicken wings*

Steps:

1. Coat chicken wings with Mandarin Glaze. Sprinkle Traeger Beef Chicken Rub onto wings. Marinate for 30 minutes or more.

2. Start the traeger and set the temperature to 350°F when ready to cook. Lid locked, 10 to 15 minutes preheat.

3. Cook the wings for 30 minutes, or up to 165°F indoor temperature.

61. ARTICHOKE & SPINACH DIP

PREP TIME: 20 Minutes

COOK TIME: 1 Hour

SERVES: 6 - 8 People

Get the football party started with a favorite of Andrew "McLovin" Perloff, from The Dan Patrick Show. Serve this creamy, smoky and savory dip with lightly grilled pita bread or smoked chips for a touchdown appetizer.

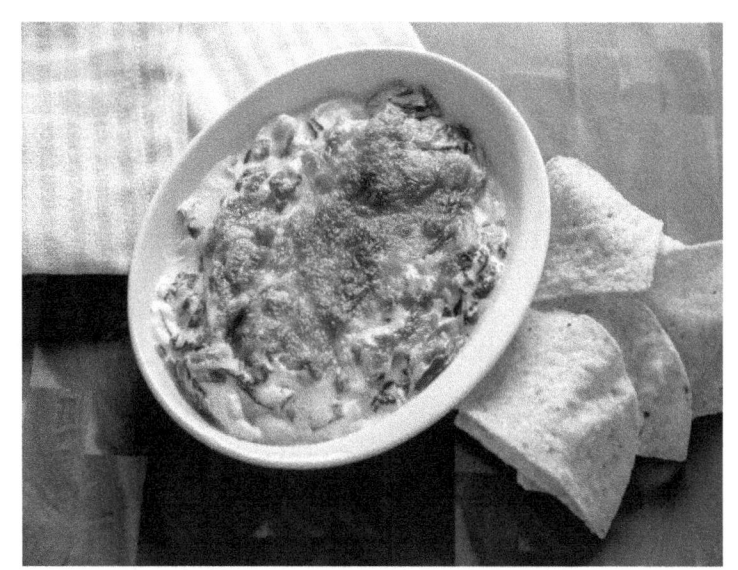

Ingredients:

- *6 Large Artichokes*
- *2 Clove Garlic, grated or diced*
- *2 Tablespoons extra-virgin olive oil*
- *1 teaspoon lemon juice*
- *To Taste salt*
- *10 Ounces Frozen Spinach, Packaged, Thawed and Drained*
- *2 Tablespoons Butter, unsalted*
- *1 Medium Shallot, finely chopped*
- *3/4 teaspoon paprika*
- *8 Ounces cream cheese*
- *1 cup heavy cream*
- *1 teaspoon salt*

- *1/2 teaspoon freshly ground black pepper*
- *1 cup mozzarella cheese*
- *1/4 cup Parmesan cheese, grated*

Steps:

1. Start the Traeger and heat the barbecue to 500°F. Lid locked, preheat 10 to 15 minutes.
2. Cut stem and top third off any artichokes — garlic in the center in between several leaves. Stir in olive oil, orange juice and butter.
3. Put artichokes on the grill directly and roast for 45 to 60 minutes.
4. Once the artichoke has cooked and softened, remove it from the grill and reduce the grill temperature to 350°F. Let cool artichokes.
5. Next, cut the core of the artichoke. Drop the leaves and peel off. Scrape the fuzzy surface of the neck and discard it with a knife. The nucleus of the artichoke must stay. Split into bits and put back.
6. Squeeze the moisture out of the spinach with cool dishtowel or towels as much as possible.
7. Melt butter over medium heat in a wide pan and sauté the shallot for 3–5 minutes until tender. Stir in the paprika and cook for about 30 seconds until fragrant.
8. Top with lettuce, artichoke, cream cheese, cream, salt and pepper. Cook, stir until warmed and reduce slightly for 8–10 minutes. Place mozzarella and parmesan in an ovenproof bakery.
9. Put bakery in the grill and warm until all the cheese is melted. Remove and add more seasoned parmesan cheese.
10. When ready to eat, remove from the grill and serve with brown bits, crackers, and pita chips.

62. SMOKED DRY RUB WINGS

PREP TIME: 15 Minutes

COOK TIME: 1 Hour

SERVES: 4 - 6 People

Most wing recipes have you swimming in sauce, but these dry rubbed wings are a healthier alternative that cut the mess, but not the flavor.

Ingredients:

- *1/4 cup salt*
- *1/4 cup brown sugar*
- *4 cups water*
- *4 Clove garlic, crushed*
- *1 teaspoon dried thyme*
- *1 Tablespoon red pepper flakes*
- *2 Pound chicken wings*
- *1/4 cup brown sugar*
- *1/2 teaspoon granulated onion*
- *1/4 teaspoon ancho or chipotle chile pepper*
- *1/4 teaspoon smoked paprika*
- *1/4 teaspoon garlic powder*
- *1/4 teaspoon Traeger Rub*

Steps:

1. For brine: In a big bowl or tub, blend brine with 4 cups of water until brown sugar and salt have dissolved.

2. Add wings to the brine. Cover and place in a fridge and leave the wings 24 hours.

3. Remove the wings from the brine, clean off and remove.

4. Set traeger temperature to 180°F when preparing to cook and preheat, lid closed for 15 minutes. Using Super Smoke if necessary for optimum taste.

5. For the rub: Combine dry rub materials in a tiny pot. Cover the wings on both sides with the mixture.

6. Place the wings on the grill and smoke for 60–90 minutes. Remove from the BBQ.

7. Rise to 450°F grill and preheat, lid closed 15 minutes. Place the wings on the grill again and cook on each side for around 3–5 minutes or until the wings are golden brown with some minor snap.

8. Remove the wings from the grill and eat as soon as possible.

63. HONEY LIME CHICKEN ADOBO SKEWERS

PREP TIME: 15 Minutes

COOK TIME: 15 Minutes

SERVES: 6 - 8 People

These adobo skewers are soaked in zestful flavor — just sauce them and let them chill out overnight, then grill them hot and fast tomorrow for a quick lunch or dinner.

Ingredients:

- *4 Chicken Breast, Diced*
- *1 Tablespoon vegetable oil*
- *2 teaspoon garlic, minced*
- *2 teaspoon onion powder*
- *3/4 cup Rice Vinegar*
- *1/4 cup soy sauce*
- *3 Tablespoon honey*

- *2 Whole lime, juiced*
- *As Needed salt*
- *As Needed black pepper*
- *8 Traeger Skewers*

Steps:

1. In a wide bowl, combine all the ingredients, including the meat.
2. Cover the mix and cool overnight.
3. Set the Traeger to high and preheat, lid shut for 15 minutes until ready to cook.
4. Place the marinated chicken on the skewers and grill it on the Traeger, rotating often until cooked (12–15 min).
5. Serve with limes grilled.

64. ROASTED HASSELBACK POTATOES

PREP TIME: 30 Minutes

COOK TIME: 2 Hours

SERVES: 6 - 8 People

Make a meal out of these potatoes. Bacon and butter are loaded into Hasselback style potatoes, slow-roasted and topped with melted cheddar cheese and fresh scallions.

Ingredients:

- *6 Large russet potatoes*
- *1 Pound bacon*
- *1/2 cup butter*

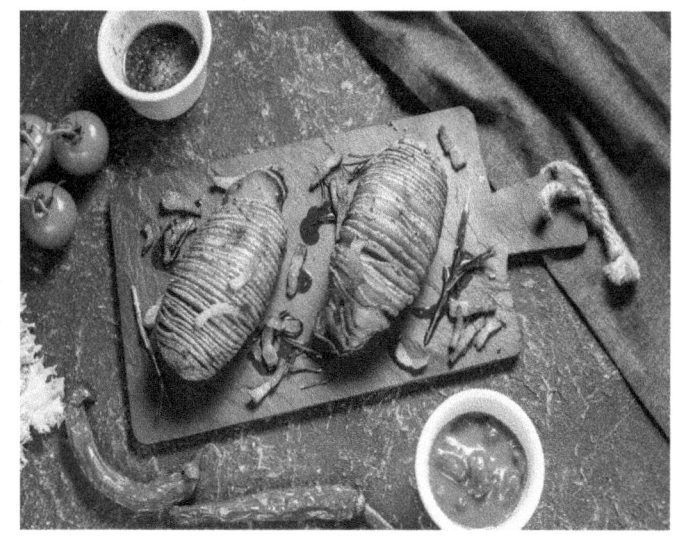

- *To Taste salt*
- *To Taste black pepper*
- *1 cup cheddar cheese*
- *3 Whole scallions*

Steps:

1. Place two wooden spoons on either side of the potato to cut the potatoes (this stops the knife from passing through all the way). Cut the potato into thin slices, leaving around 1/4" on the edges.
2. Then break bacon slices into tiny parts about the size of a stamp. Place them in the cracks between each slice.
3. In a broad cast-iron skillet, put the potato. Top the potatoes with hard butter slices (and, if desired, thin slivers of cold butter may also be placed between the potato slices)—salt and pepper season.
4. Set the traeger to 350°F and preheat, lid closed for 15 minutes when ready to cook.
5. Put the cast iron on the grill directly and cook for 2 hours. Top potatoes with more butter and grind every 30 minutes with melted butter.
6. Sprinkle with cheddar and return to grill to melt for the last 10 minutes of cooking.
7. Top with chives or scallions to finish.

65. BAKED VENISON TATER TOT CASSEROLE

PREP TIME: 10 Minutes

COOK TIME: 40 Minutes

SERVES: 4 - 6 People

You'll go wild for these tots. Wood-fired tater tots, hearty ground venison, creamy mushroom soup and peas make for the ultimate comfort dish when you're hankering for a homestyle meal.

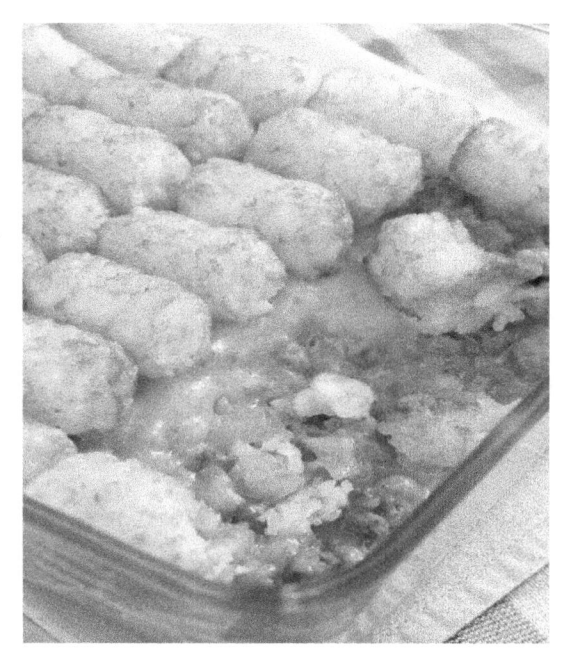

Ingredients:

- *2 Pound Venison, ground*
- *2 Can Peas, canned*
- *2 Can Cream Mushroom Soup*
- *28 Ounce Tater Tots, Frozen*

Steps:

1. Cook ground venison in a medium-high skillet until browned. Drain extra fat and put venison aside.
2. Combine venison, peas and soup in a 13x9 pan. Top with the tots of the tater.
3. Set the traeger to 350°F and preheat, lid closed for 15 minutes until ready to cook.
4. Place the casserole directly on the grill and cook for 30 minutes. Serve hot, yes!

66. BAKED GARLIC PARMESAN WINGS

PREP TIME: 15 Minutes

COOK TIME: 30 Minutes

SERVES: 4 - 6 People

If you're looking for simple and downright delicious, these wings are calling your name. Chicken Rub seasoned wings are grilled and topped with parmesan cheese and fresh parsley for some handheld happiness.

Ingredients:

- *1/2 cup Traeger Chicken Rub*
- *5 Pounds chicken wings*
- *1 cup butter*
- *10 Clove garlic, minced*
- *2 Tablespoons Traeger Chicken Rub*
- *1 cup Parmesan cheese, grated*
- *3 Tablespoons parsley, chopped*

Steps:

1. Set the temperature to maximum when about to cook and preheat, lid shut for 15 minutes. Set to 500°F if necessary for better performance.

2. Toss the wings in a wide bowl with 1/2 cup of Traeger Chicken Rub.

3. Barbecue and simmer for 10 minutes. Simmer on barbecue. Flip wings and simmer for another 10 minutes. Test the internal wing temperature and the temperature needed is 165–180°F.

4. To produce the garlic sauce: When the chicken is cooked, mix in a medium-sized bowl butter, garlic and remaining rub and roast on a pan over medium heat. Heat sauce, stirring regularly for 8–10 minutes.

5. Once the wings are fried, take off the grill and put them in a wide bowl —apply the garlic sauce, the parmesan cheese and the parsley to the wings. Serve and enjoy!

67. TRAEGER SHRIMP

PREP TIME: 15 Minutes

COOK TIME: 10 Minutes

SERVES: 8 - 12 People

Bring the island vibes to your backyard with Dennis The Prescott's Traeger jerk shrimp recipe. Homemade jerk seasoning and zesty lime add a bold Caribbean kick to your favorite shellfish.

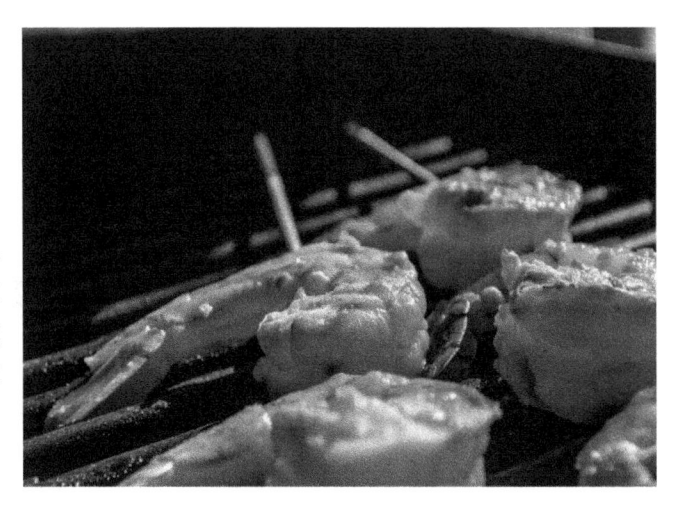

Ingredients:

- *1 Tablespoon brown sugar*
- *1 Tablespoon smoked paprika*
- *1 teaspoon garlic powder*
- *1/4 teaspoon Thyme, ground*
- *1/4 teaspoon ground cayenne pepper*
- *1 teaspoon sea salt*
- *1 lime zest*
- *2 Pounds Shrimp, in shell*
- *3 Tablespoons olive oil*

Steps:

1. In a shallow pot, add herbs, salt and lime zest and blend. Place the shrimp in a big bowl, then drizzle with the olive oil, apply the spice mixture and blend to make sure that every shrimp is covered.

2. Set the temperature to 450°F when preparing to cook and preheat, lid closed for 15 minutes

3. Place the shrimp on the grill and cook it on each side for 2–3 minutes until solid, translucent and fried.

4. Serve with lime wedges, fresh cilantro, mint, and Caribbean Hot Pepper Sauce. Enjoy!

68. GRILLED FRUIT SKEWERS WITH YOGURT SAUCE

PREP TIME: 30 Minutes

COOK TIME: 6 Minutes

SERVES: 2 - 4 People

This Christmas fruit recipe has a dash of spice & a hint of smoke. Serve it for your sweet holiday side dish or as an appetizer.

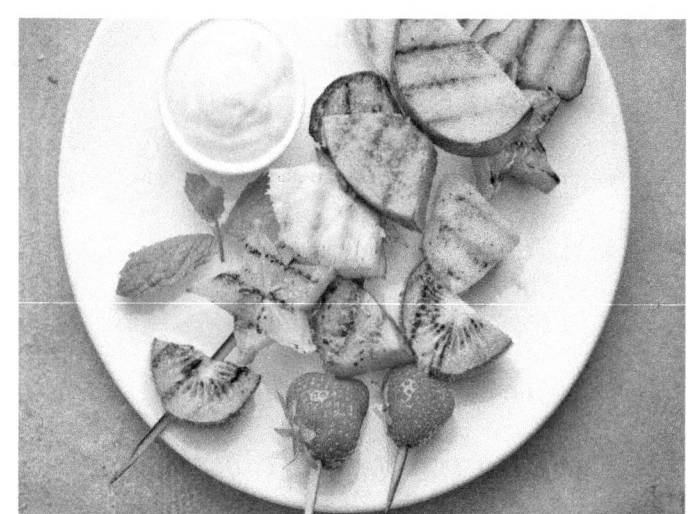

Ingredients:

- *1/4 cup water*
- *1/2 cup brown sugar*
- *1 teaspoon ground cinnamon*
- *1/2 orange, juiced*
- *1 Apple, green*
- *2 Nectarines*
- *1 Persimmon*
- *8 Ounce Yogurt, vanilla*
- *1/2 orange, juiced*

Steps:

1. Soak them in water for at least 30 minutes if you use wooden skewers.

2. Combine brown sugar with 1/4 cup of water, cinnamon and orange zest in a small pot. Bring to a boil in medium heat. Remove from heat and hold at room temperature to cool.

3. Set the Traeger to 275°F when preparing to cook and preheat, lid shut down 15 minutes.

4. Cut the fruit into 1-inch pieces and thread 2 parts of each type of fruit on each skewer.

5. Grill the skewer until the fruit is moist and charred softly around 6 minutes, rotating the sprouts every 1-1/2 minutes.

6. Make sure the brown sugar syrup is brushed after every turn.

7. Make the dipping sauce while the fruit is grilling. In a serving bowl, whisk the yogurt, orange juice and 1 tablespoon of the brown sugar syrup.

8. Place the skewers on a plate and eat with the dipping sauce.

69. GRILLED OYSTERS BY JOURNEY SOUTH

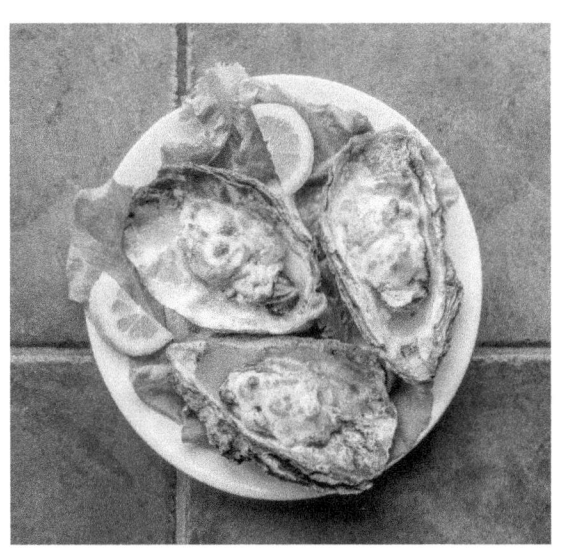

PREP TIME: 20 Minutes

COOK TIME: 30 Minutes

SERVES: 4 - 6 People

Nail National Oyster Day with this recipe from Journey South. Start with a sautéed mixture of onion, bell peppers, garlic, and lemon juice. Add in some Traeger Chicken Rub and white wine and let this sauce make those oysters sing.

Ingredients:

- *2 Medium onion*
- *1 Medium Bell Pepper, Red*
- *5 Tablespoons extra-virgin olive oil*
- *2 lemons*
- *3 teaspoons dried thyme*
- *3 Bay Leaves, dried*
- *5 Tablespoons garlic, minced*
- *3 Tablespoons Traeger Chicken Rub*
- *3 Tablespoons Worcestershire sauce*
- *5 Tablespoons Hot Pepper Sauce*
- *1/4 cup Wine, white*
- *4 Butter, Sticks*
- *12 Whole Oysters, shucked*
- *As Needed Italian Cheese Blend*

Steps:

1. Set the grill temperature strong when preparing to cook and preheat, cover closed for 15 minutes.
2. Preheat olive oil over medium heat in cast iron skillet. Cut onion and bell peppers and place them into a preheated skillet.
3. Juice lemons in the saucepan. In the Traeger Chicken Rub, add thyme, bay leaves, garlic and blend.
4. Cook the carrots until they are transparent and peppers have soften for 5–7 minutes.
5. Add butter and spicy sauce to Worcestershire. Add white wine and four butter sticks. Sauté 15 more minutes.

6. When the sauce cooks, rinse the oysters and turn and drop them at the bottom of the sell.

7. Put the oysters on Traeger and finish with the sauce. Five minutes of prep time.

8. Finish with and eat with Italian cheese.

70. DOUBLE-DECKER PULLED PORK NACHOS WITH SMOKED CHEESE

PREP TIME: 5 Minutes

COOK TIME: 55 Minutes

SERVES: 4 - 6 People

Traeger Pulled Pork Nachos taste so good, and we stack them twice. More smoked cheese, more mouthwatering pulled pork, and more of your favorite toppings in every delicious bite.

Ingredients:

- *8 Ounce Cheese, pepper jack*
- *8 Ounce Cheese, sharp cheddar*
- *As Needed Tortilla Chips*
- *2 cup Pork, pulled, leftover*
- *As Needed black olives*
- *As Needed jalapeño, diced*
- *As Needed cilantro*

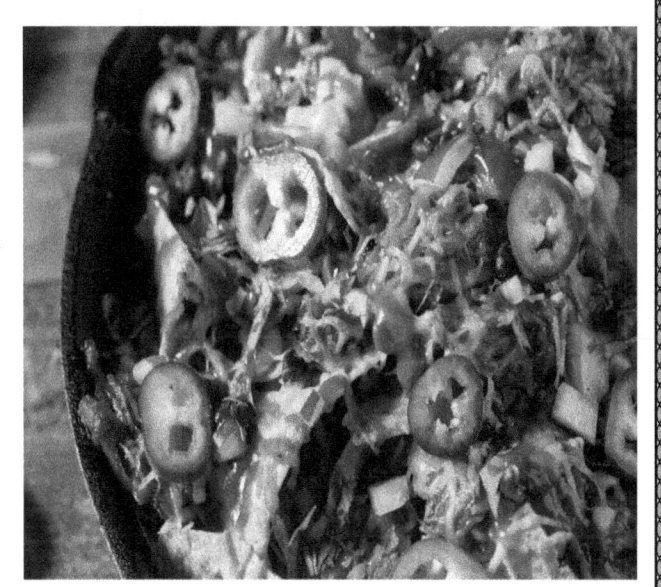

Steps:

1. Start the Traeger and set the temperature at 165°F when you are ready to cook. Preheat for 10–15 minutes with the lid closed.

2. Put the cheese (frozen) on a rack over an ice-filled tray. Maybe you want to cut the cheese into smaller portions, perhaps 2 or 3 chunks per block, so that it smokes faster.

3. For 45 to 60 minutes, smoke the cheeses; cool. Cut cheeses (approximately 1 cup each) and set aside.

4. Turn heat up to 350°F on Traeger and preheat, lid closed, 10-15 minutes.

5. Place the chips on a broad baker and apply the grilled and smoked cheeses equally. On the grill, place the bakery sheet and cook for about 10 minutes, or until the cheese is melted and blubbly.

6. Take the pan from the Traeger and begin putting the nachos on the double sheet. Assemble the nachos on the bottom with a sheet of cheesy chips, pulled pork and more cheesy chips. Fill it with your own nacho toppings. Eat warm.

71. BAKED PICKLES WITH BUTTERMILK DIP

PREP TIME: 20 Minutes

COOK TIME: 10 Minutes

SERVES: 4 - 6 People

These pickles are the ultimate game day appetizer. They're breaded in a delicious blend of spices and panko, baked, and paired with a creamy buttermilk dip you won't be able to get enough of.

Ingredients:

- *1 (16 oz) jar dill pickle spears*
- *2 large egg*

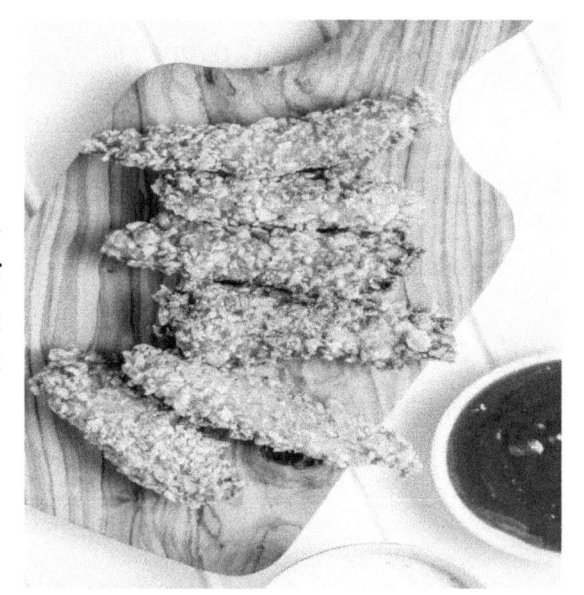

- *1/3 cup all-purpose flour*
- *1 teaspoon hot sauce*
- *1/2 teaspoon chipotle chile powder*
- *1/2 teaspoon anchochile powder*
- *1/2 teaspoon dried oregano*
- *1/4 teaspoon Jacobsen Salt Co. Pure Kosher Sea Salt*
- *1/4 teaspoon black pepper*
- *1 cup panko breadcrumbs*
- *1/2 cup Parmesan cheese, grated*
- *1/2 cup mayonnaise*
- *2 Tablespoon buttermilk*
- *1 teaspoon fresh chopped parsley*
- *1/2 teaspoon Jacobsen Salt Co. Pure Kosher Sea Salt*
- *1/4 teaspoon garlic powder*
- *1/4 teaspoon garlic salt*
- *1/4 teaspoon onion powder*
- *1/4 teaspoon black pepper*

Steps:

1. Set temperature to 450°F when preparing to cook and preheat, lid closed for 15 minutes.
2. Place a cooling rack on the top of a bakery sheet and spray the rack with oil.
3. Drop the pickles, scatter over towels of paper and pat off.
4. Add milk, flour, hot sauce, chili powders, oregano, garlic powder, salt, pipes and sweep to blend in a small bowl.

5. Combine the breadcrumbs and Parmesan in a wide bowl.

6. Put the pickles into the egg blend, remove, let the excess drop out and pass it into the breadcrumb blend. Toss to cover.

7. Move the pickle to the fitted cooling rack and position in a single row.

8. Place the bakery directly on the grill and cook until the pickles are crisp and golden brown, around 10 minutes

9. Combine all the ingredients of the dip in a blender and mix until they are smooth. Season with salt and pepper to match

72. ALDER SMOKED SCALLOPS WITH CITRUS & GARLIC BUTTER SAUCE

PREP TIME: 15 Minutes

COOK TIME: 35 Minutes

SERVES: 4 - 6 People

Scallops are quick and easy to smoke; this citrus and garlic glaze will make this summer meal over the top amazing. Alder is the preferred wood pellet for any meat, so make sure you have it handy for any Traeger recipe.

Ingredients:

- *2 Pounds sizeable dry sea scallops*
- *Kosher salt*
- *Freshly ground black pepper*
- *8 Tablespoons salted butter, melted*
- *1 Clove garlic, minced*
- *1 Small orange*

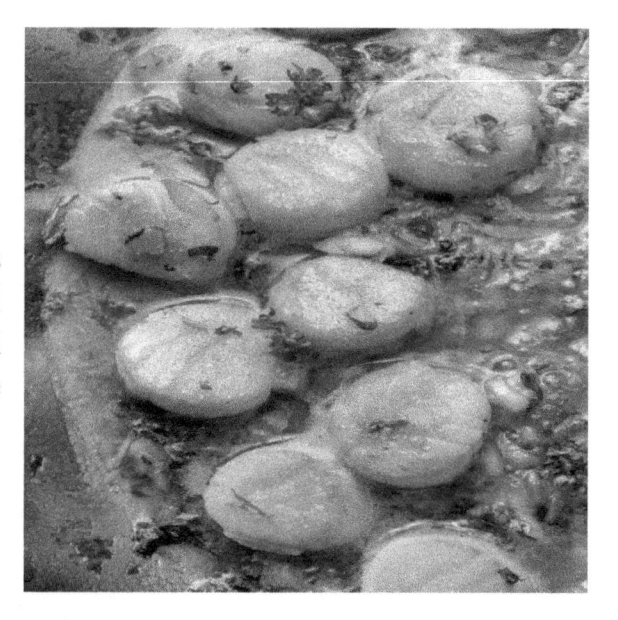

- *1/4 teaspoon Worcestershire sauce*
- *1 1/2 teaspoon fresh chopped parsley or tarragon*
- *Flat-leaf parsley, for serving*

Steps:

1. Wash scallops under cool running spray and dry them completely with paper towels. Remove all tags of the abductor muscle on the sides of the scallops.

2. Arrange the scallops on a cooling plate and season with salt and pepper.

3. Level Traeger temperature to 165°F when ready to cook and preheat, lid closed for 15 minutes. Using Super Smoke if necessary for optimum taste.

4. Place the baking sheet on the grill with the scallops, smoke for 20 minutes.

5. Create your sauce as your scallops are smoking. In a small cup, melt the butter over medium-low flame. Apply a tablespoon of salt, garlic, Worcestershire, part of the orange zest and juice, and parsley. Simmer 5 minutes.

6. Take from the grill the bakery layer and set away. Increase to 400°F and preheat with lid closed. Optional: Pre-heat in the grill with an oyster bed or an oyster tray. Such giant iron pans are a perfect place to cook the scallops.

7. Return the bakery sheet to the grill with the skillet, brown the butter sauce and reserve for serving. Roast until tender and smooth, 10 to 15 minutes. The period depends on the size of the scallops. Do not overcook. If you use an oyster bowl, lightly brush each compartment with olive oil to prevent sticking. Spoon the butter sauce over each of the scallops, and save for eating.

8. Serve the scallops soft with a little bit of orange peel, fresh parsley, and the sauce with moist citrus fruits and garlic butter.

73. COLD SMOKED CHEESE

PREP TIME: 5 Minutes

COOK TIME: 2 Hours

SERVES: 8 - 12 People

Infuse rich hardwood flavor into your cheese of choice by cold smoking it on the Traeger. Pair with crackers, wine, or pickled vegetables for the perfect snack.

Ingredients:

- *Preferred kind of block cheese: Mozzarella, provolone, cheddar*

Steps:

1. Set the Traeger temperature at 165°F when ready to cook and close the lid for 15 minutes to preheat.

2. Place a half-size bowl in the middle of a big bowl. Surround half-size bowl with ice to the top.

3. Place the cheese on top of toothpicks or a cooling rack in the half-size pan so that it can move around, avoiding sticking — place the pot on the grill.

4. 1 hour smoke cheese. Open the grill and turn over the cheese. Add more ice to the melted water and smoke for another hour.

5. Remove from the grill and wrap it in paper parchment. Place in the refrigerator and allow to set for 2 to 3 days. This allows the flavor to soften.

6. After 2 to 3 days, unwrap, slice and eat your favorite cracker, snacked veggies and wine from the refrigerator.

74. TANDOORI CHICKEN WINGS

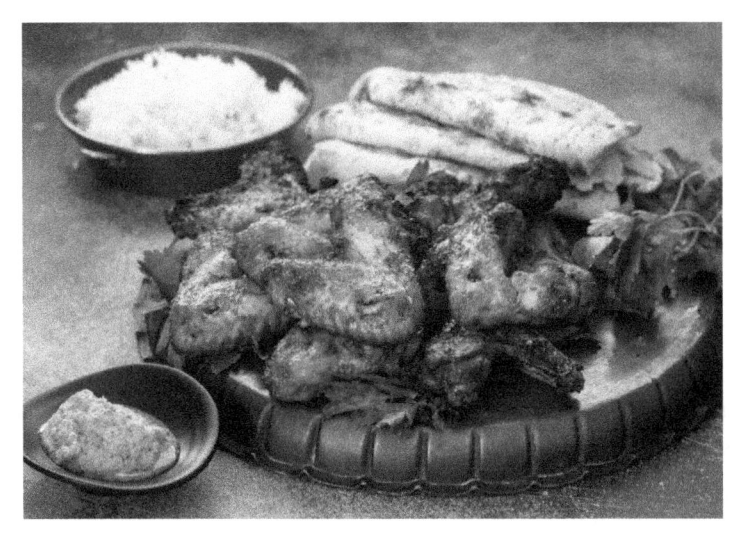

PREP TIME: 30 Minutes

COOK TIME: 50 Minutes

SERVES: 4 - 6 People

Indian spices and flavors do not get the spotlight that they deserve. The exotic tastes of India are deliciously developed, intoxicatingly fragrant and heart-warming and as spicy as you want to make them.

Ingredients:

- *1/4 cup Yogurt*
- *1 Whole Scallions, minced*
- *1 Tablespoon minced cilantro leaves*
- *2 teaspoons ginger, minced*
- *1 teaspoon Masala*
- *1 teaspoon salt*
- *1 teaspoon ground black pepper*
- *1 1/2 Pound chicken wings*
- *1/4 cup Yogurt*
- *2 Tablespoons mayonnaise*
- *2 Tablespoons Cucumber*
- *2 teaspoons lemon juice*
- *1/2 teaspoon cumin*

- *1/2 teaspoon salt*
- *1/8 teaspoon cayenne pepper*

Steps:

1. In a mixer jar, mix yogurt, skallions, coriander, ginger, garam masala, salt and pepper and process until smooth. Pour over the chicken and rub all the wings with the mixture. Cool for 4 to 8 hours. Remove wings from excess marinade; dump marinade.

2. Set the temperature to 350°F and preheat, lid closed, 10-15 minutes when ready to cook. Brush the grill with oil.

3. Place the wings on the grill. Cook for 45 to 50 minutes, or until the skin is dark and crisp and the beef is not pink at the bone any more. During the frying, switch once or twice to stop the wings from sticking to the grill.

4. Combine all the ingredients for the sauce; set aside and cool before ready to eat.

5. When fried, switch to a pan or pot. When done, serve with sauce of yogurt.

75. ROASTED JALAPENO CHEDDAR DEVILED EGGS

PREP TIME: 10 Minutes

COOK TIME: 30 Minutes

SERVES: 6 - 8 People

Don't wait until Easter for deviled eggs. These spicy roasted jalapeno deviled eggs are an excellent appetizer for a family party or while watching the game.

Ingredients:

- *7 Eggs, hard-boiled*
- *3 Tablespoon mayonnaise*
- *1 teaspoon brown mustard*
- *1 teaspoon apple cider vinegar*
- *1 Dash hot sauce*
- *1 jalapeño pepper, seeded and minced*
- *To Taste salt and pepper*
- *1/2 cup shredded cheddar cheese*
- *To Taste paprika*

Steps:

1. Start your Traeger and set it to 180°F (80°C). Preheat, 10–15 minutes lid locked.
2. Place your eggs on the grill directly and smoke for 30 minutes.
3. Remove from the grill and cool the eggs. Smoking the eggs brings a mildly yellowed colour to them, with a good smoky flavor. If you prefer a classic white egg, skip this move.
4. Cut the eggs in the longitudinal direction and scoop the egg yolks into a gallon zipper bag.

5. Put mayo, mustard, vinegar, hot sauce, roast jalapeños and salt and pepper into your container.

6. Loop the bag closed and knead all the ingredients together with your hands until absolutely smooth.

7. Squeeze the yolk mixture into one corner and break off the end. In the whites, add the yolk mixture.

8. Sprinkle with thinly sliced cheddar or paprika and cool before ready to eat.

76. GARLIC PARMESAN CHICKEN WINGS

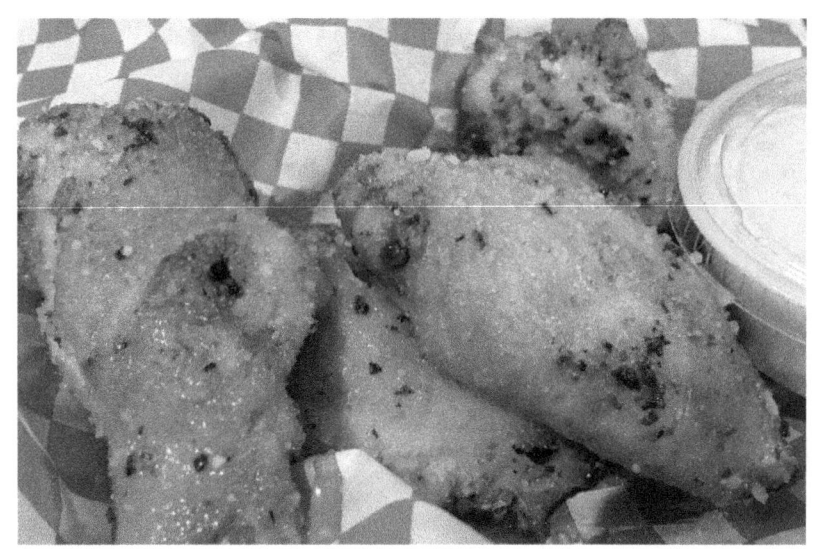

PREP TIME: 10 Minutes

COOK TIME: 25 Minutes

SERVES: 4 - 6 People

Give your wings some garlic butter love. These wings are grilled, tossed in a flavorful sauce and topped with melt-in-your-mouth fresh grated parmesan.

Ingredients:

- *3 lbs Pound chicken wings*
- *As Needed Meat Church Gourmet Garlic and Herb Seasoning*
- *1 Stick unsalted butter*
- *12 Clove garlic, minced*
- *As Needed Parmesan cheese, grated*
- *As Needed parsley, chopped*

Steps:

1. Start the Traeger with grill directions when ready to cook. Set the heat to 450°F (500°F, if Wi-Fi enabled) and preheat, lid shut down for 10 to 15 minutes.

2. When you have purchased the entire wing, remove the tip and separate the drummettes and wing. Pat them dry. Season the wings with Meat Church Gourmet Garlic & Herb seasoning generously on both sides.

3. For the butter with garlic: heat the butter in a small cup. Add the minced garlic and cook for 5 minutes until perfumed. Disable and restart.

4. With a cumulative cook period of 20 minutes, place the wings directly on your Traeger cooking grill. Flip the wings halfway of the cook. I like to have as many tasty bits of charcoal on my wings and tossing them would aid on each side.

5. Chicken wings will hit 165–180°F internal temperature after 20 minutes. Although chicken is healthy to consume at 165°F, cooking wings is all right because it is difficult to dry it.

6. Toss the wings in the sauce with garlic oil. Put them 5 minutes in your Traeger so the sauce can be mounted. Remove from the BBQ.

7. When the wings are dry, grate Parmesan cheese over the wings. Garnish parsley. Enjoy the ranch or by yourself.

THE 9 BEST PELLET GRILLS REVIEWED

1. THE BEST ALL-AROUND PELLET SMOKER — CAMP CHEF SMOKEPRO SG24 WIFI PELLET GRILL

The Camp Chef Smoke PRO SG24 is a fantastic mid-size smoker who finds a perfect balance between consistency and dollar worth.

Camp Chef has recently released its new Gen 2 PID controller, which gives you excellent temperature control and the ability to exactly control your desired smoke.

You can easily fit several ribs racks on one occasion with 429 square inches of cooking area (plus a 382 square inch rack). Unlike a charcoal smoker, in 10 minutes you'll be up and running.

If you need more space, you can upgrade to our high-end pick-up, the SmokePro SGX model, which allows you to work with 1236 square centimeters.

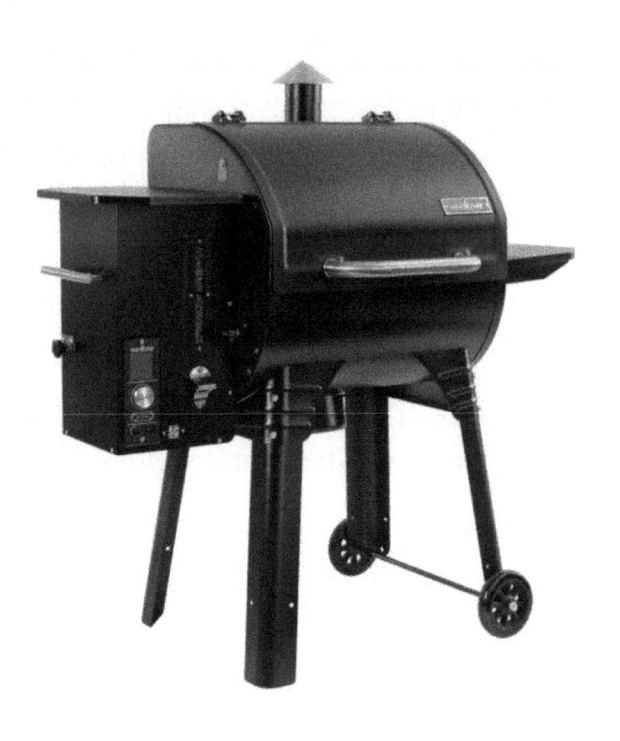

The SG24 ticks all the pellet grill boxes at this medium price point. You will enjoy the setting and you will forget the style of cooking with two meat samples, clean smoke flavor, and minimal cleaning ash.

The latest model also includes wireless Internet access, so you can monitor and control your grill on your telephone. All the key components are made of strong weighing stainless steel and look durable. You can choose between 160-500°F and dial the exact smoke of 1–10.

You should pass over a plate when you need more fuel to cook, so that the fire from the fireplace seeds the food at temperatures up to 650°F.

What we liked:

- Smokestack location — The camp chef has put the smokestack on the rear of the building, allowing you more space for research on the right-hand side.

- Easy cleaning — You may not know how much cleanup is needed if you haven't used many smokers before. This machine includes a trap door to clean the pot easily.

- Efficient consumption of pellets — we are always surprised how few pellets this unit eats. Your results may vary, however, depending on the weather.

- Searing capability — Most pellet smokers are struggling to sear, so this option is great, especially when you want to barbecue a lot of steaks and burgers.

What we didn't like:

- Occasional temperature sensor quality management issues — while it doesn't appear to concern everybody, certain users encounter a temperature sensor problem after a few applications. Camp Chef has outstanding help, though, and they will be easy to fix should any problems occur.

- The code can be slow and has minimal features — there were a number of issues with low performance and accessibility at the time of cooking.

The software needs to provide patches, and we trust that Camp Chef tackles these problems. They ought to remember that without the program, you will not use the grill perfectly (when you have modified the firmware), this will be a deal-breaker because the software experience is important to you.

We have had trouble seeking anything else to blame this bbq. This is a super flexible device, especially with the sear box connect.

You can't go wrong with this unit if you are concerned about buying a charcoal smoker and only shooting it 3 or 4 times a year. You're going to search for some reason to shoot it and play with smoking.

SmokePro SG24 is available for free delivery on the Camp Chef page in Black and Bronze.

2. RUNNER UP — TRAEGER PRO 575 WOOD PELLET GRILL

If your budget is extendable and you want the leading brand with all the new technology, the Traeger Pro is a perfect choice.

While Traeger has recently been fashionable, they made a range of changes in the Pro models in 2019, which render it worthy of consideration. The Pro also offers Wi-Fi for remote access and grill tracking.

The latest Pro also fixes a variety of typical issues with older Traegers. Reduced heating level and temperature control complexity. A brushless DC engine is used for the new D2 direct drive to produce higher torque at a lower RPM. What does this mean? The motor will transform the pellet auger quicker, enabling you to heat the fireplace quicker and hotter.

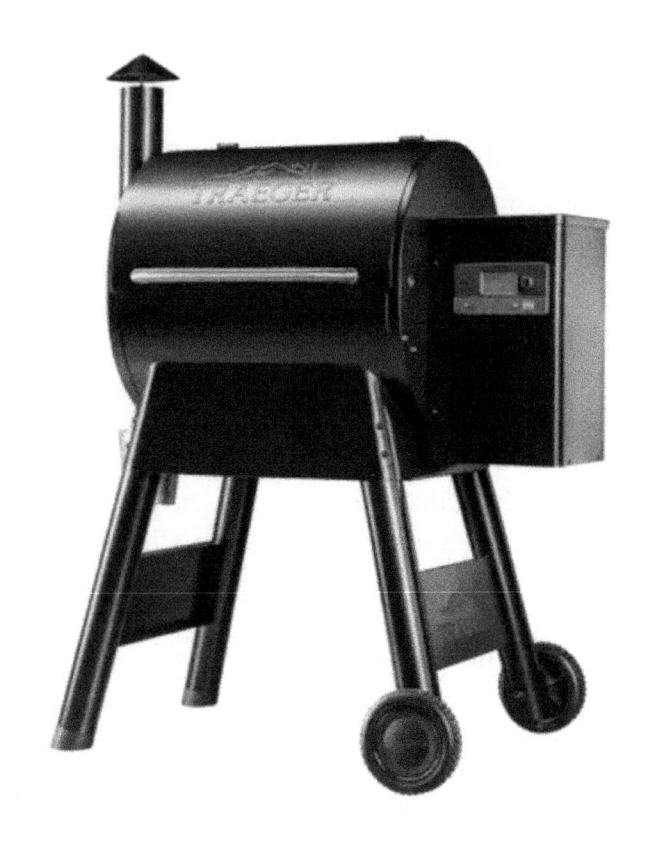

These features only come with the top of the Timberline range and, in our view, make the Pro a great buy. For either 575 or 780 square inches of cooking area, you may pick the Pro. The additional room would save you a mere $200, but remember how many individuals you need to cater with, this may be a place that you might save more money. You can also choose between color schemes in black or bronze. You receive a temperature sensor that allows your food temperature to be monitored from the grill or via the Traeger app.

What we like:

- Highly accurate D2 PID controller — The Traeger Pro controller uses a variable speed fan that can speed up or slow down to reach and hold a more exact temperature. You can set the temperature within 5°F increments.

- WiFi connectivity — The so-called WiFIRE technology is quite smart, allowing you to control temperatures and monitor your food from anywhere via your smartphone.

You can even choose from hundreds of pre-programmed recipes, which will control the entire cooking cycle, changing the temperature and air circulation for you.

What we don't like:

- Essential accessories pay an additional $149.98 for the grill cover & sliding shelf ($19.98 on 575 models).

- The Pro series represents a nice option of interest to get results with the Traeger collection, aside from needing to fork out extra for shelf and cover.

A quick warning word. Traeger marginally modified their 2019 product naming procedure. The older models are called Pro 34, whereby the 34 is the height of the principal grill bar.

The new versions using the whole cooking surface on their behalf. You may save some money on one of our older versions, if you don't think you'll take advantage of the WiFi functionality, however, in our opinion, the updated drivetrain, engine, and fan plus WiFi make the Pro Series our runner up to the best pellet grill.

3. THE BEST BUDGET PELLET GRILL — Z GRILLS ZPG-7002E WOOD PELLET GRILL & SMOKER

It is still hard to suggest a pellet grill for the budget. When so much development is involved, there is even more that can fail (or, to start with, never function properly).

When we learned that Z Grills rendered Traeger standard grills at drastically cheaper costs, we were fascinated. The business claims to have arisen suddenly, but for many years now they have been producing grills out of China for other US companies, including Traeger. They appeared to have agreed to bypass the broker and started marketing their products directly to the public in 2017. The Pit Boss 700FB or the Traeger Pro 575 will be the nearest competitor with 700 square inches of cooking surface (divided into 500" main and 200" small grass) and 20-pound hopper.

But with the Z-Grill, the Traeger is similar at a substantially lower price, although there is no accompanying app.

The simplest variant is 7002E. You may choose a 700E package, which has a handy cabinet for holding pellets or BBQ devices if you choose to pay a little extra.

What we like:

- Money value – Getting a pellet barbeque with this hopper size and a lot of cooking space is already good for the price. Throw in solid stainless steel; the digital temperature and pellet control system was newly updated in 2019, and the Z-grill starts to look like a steal.

- Generous 3-year contract – The extended coverage is important as it is a fresh product, and we haven't seen how far it works. 3 years are on par with more costly brands but with the Pit Boss less than five years.

What we don't like:

- Cleaning unused pellets — it can be tough to clear some unused pellets from the hopper unless you decide to adjust the pellet form. To do this, you may need to invest in a small vacuum.

- No insulation blanket — you can purchase an insulation blanket for the Traeger that is helpful while cooking under 40°F at outside temperatures.

- Few individuals who had trouble with an inadequate temperature control device have already been identified. This seems to have been a concern since it came out in 2019 when the software was revised.

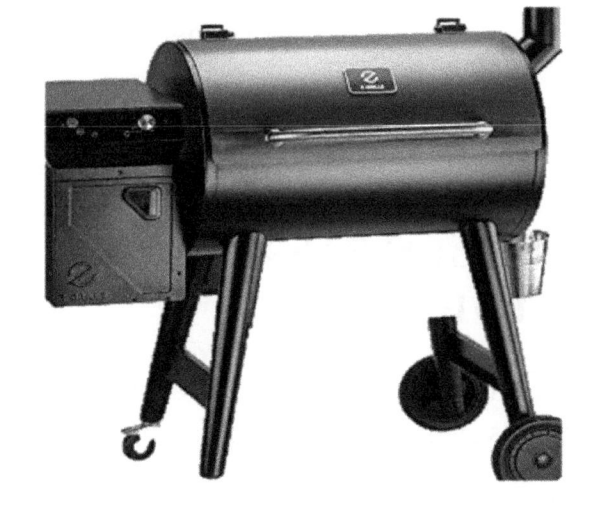

If you don't mind the fact that you purchase from a new Chinese brand, the Z-grill 7002 is the strongest budget pellet barbecue on the market today. So, if it helps you feel stronger, most US grill firms also do all their production in China. It looks like customer support is still quite sensitive from our study.

When we last checked out, you get a $49.90 free grill cover on your Z Grills website.

4. THE BEST PORTABLE PELLET SMOKER — GREEN MOUNTAIN GRILLS DAVY CROCKETT WIFI GRILL

The Green Mountain Grills Davy Crockett is billed as "the go-to grill for small families, campers, tailgaters, RVers, or anyone who wants to cook two racks of ribs or 4-6 nice steaks or a bunch of burgers." It is a stainless steel, pellet fed smoker/grill, and works with one App via it's own WiFi.

Green Mountain Grills makes wood pellets, but the will work well with any wood pellet so you might as well buy in bulk. With the capability of heating accurately between 200° and 550°F, (more about this later) the does a decent job as both a smoker and a grill. On top of that, it's packed with some surprisingly high tech features.

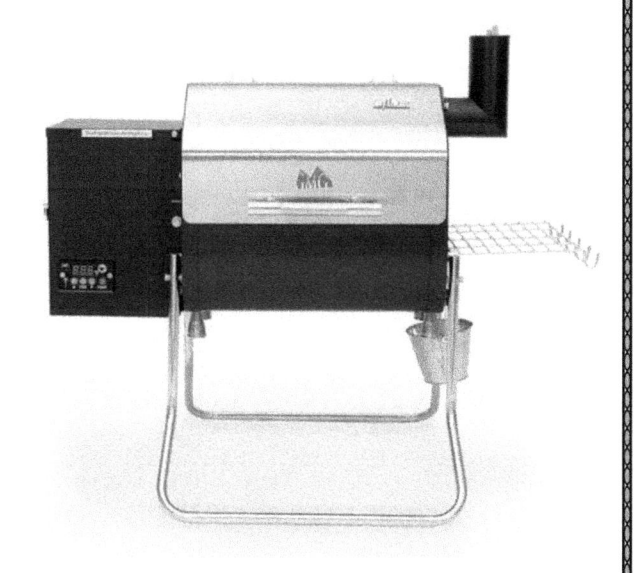

What we liked:

- Compact design — Grill is filled along with the tools that the smoker wants to bring from a range of outlets, and the pliable legs make it simple to travel.

- Accurate temperature regulation — The Davy Crockett allows you much better power than many other pellets. You will make 5-degree modifications using the manual control panel. Then, if you decide to turn it down, you can make one-off changes to the device.

- You may, for instance, schedule it to cook for 5 hours at 225°F, and then adjust it automatically for another 4 hours to 250°F.

- Clever warnings — It's also good to learn that the device does not tap into wood pellets and the temperature decreases. It is likely to go out and test the barbecue.

What we don't like:

- Uncomfortable to move with one person — because of the smoker's weight and the uncomfortable manner in which the legs get off, we still suggest two people maneuvering the smoker.

- Wi-Fi access is often inconsistent. It depends on the specific configuration, but from time to time we find that the grill would lose connectivity.

- The construction standard is outstanding, aside from this. The fabrics are voluminous and look like the last. Like other smokers you set up once and go indefinitely, this machine can be quickly folded and transferred.

You won't be able to cook as fast as certain other grill balls, but the machine will hit 420°F.

You may also prepare the perfect amount of food with a fairly limited box. A 10 lb. brisket or a couple of ribs shouldn't be an issue to satisfy campers!

5. BEST LARGE PELLET SMOKER — CAMP CHEF SMOKEPRO LUX PELLET GRILL

This is for you if you liked the sound of our best complete range Camp Chef PG24DLX, but you only needed more than 429 square inches of cooking area.

Camp Chef SmokePro LUX has a colossal 875 square inches of cooking surface and weighs 180 lbs., it's a large boy pellet barbecue. Whereas the hopper is only 18" in size, a single load in mild weather can last 12-14 hours. When the air is colder, it will take much faster.

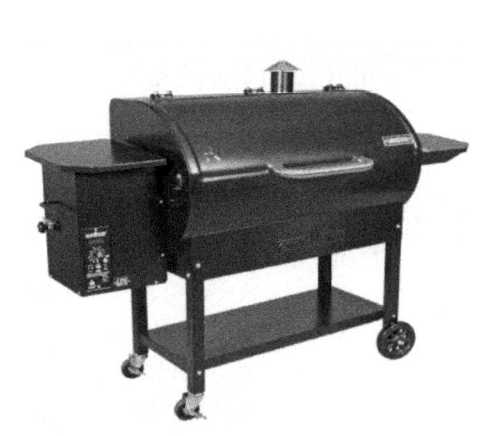

What we like:

- Big scale — The LUX has an enormous amount of room over the other versions. You will smoke a 30 lb. pork butt with two 20 lb. briskets concurrently.

- Add sear box option — With a maximum temperature of around 400°F, the grill is not great for searing. You can get around that with the extra sear pack, which includes a 16,000 BTU propane burner that can sear up to 900°F.

- Simple to clean — In comparison to other pellet grills, it's simple to clean the burned pellets' residue. Unused pellets may also be quickly separated from the hopper and auger.

What we don't like:

- Low standard beef study — the study with kinks which splits fairly quickly. Normally, we'd prescribe a professional third-party automated thermometer, but handle it with severe care if you focus on the factory report.

- Issues in synchronization — The time sensor is user-friendly, but you might run into problems when the temperature is 20-50°F off. You should drive around with your thermometer easily.

- Otherwise, the only other fault could be a little brighter with the installation instructions. That said, it should not take more than one hour, and if you watch a video installation, it is much easier.

Other pellet grills worth considering

These are the pellet grills that our main selections missed narrowly. They are always worth trying out and they may be the right option for you, based on the particular specifications.

6. CAMP CHEF WOODWIND 24 PELLET GRILL — A RELIABLE MID-SIZED OPTION

Update: Camp Chef recently revealed an upgraded Woodwind grill with an improved PID controller and wireless internet.

Two smokers from the "Smoke Pro" Camp Chef line were already included, but we couldn't leave Woodwind out of our list. This grill offers a generous cooking surface area of 570 inches and a removable top warming rack.

This is the newest model, so you can opt for a Wi-Fi version. There are also a variety of alternative setups, including a side sear box or side kick burner.

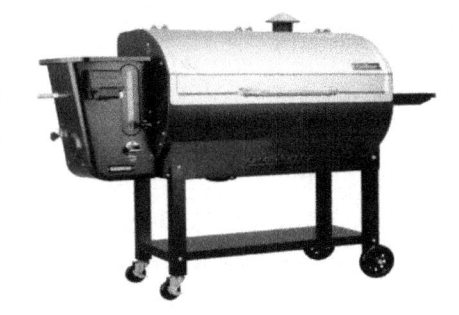

While Woodwind has several parallels with the Smoke Pro line-up, there are several noticeable variations.

They are:

- *Wi-Fi capability*

- *More extensive and improved cover on the pellet hopper*
- *Heaver legs*
- *Lower storage shelf*
- *Stainless steel lid and firepot*
- *Blue LED screen readout that's easier to see in direct sunlight*
- *The price is a step up from the DLX PG24.*

These are good choices, and the Woodwind upgrades are not a breakthrough, and the one that you choose is depending on the budget and how you can afford it when it is different.

7. REC TEC GRILLS RT-700 WI-FI ENABLED WOOD PELLET GRILL — A TREMENDOUS HIGH-END OPTION

This REC TEC grill could be included with our top choices above. REC TEC combines the precision and quality that the RT-700 offers with modern upgrades such as Wi-Fi, dual meat samples, and a better PID controller.

The knob allows you to set the temperature in 5°F intervals, a regulation degree you don't see in any of the cheaper pellet grills.

The name of the company includes the main grill area of 702 square inches. You will offer more than 1000 with an extra warming rack. This is not a budget grill, though it compares well with Traeger's more expensive Ironwood and Timberline series.

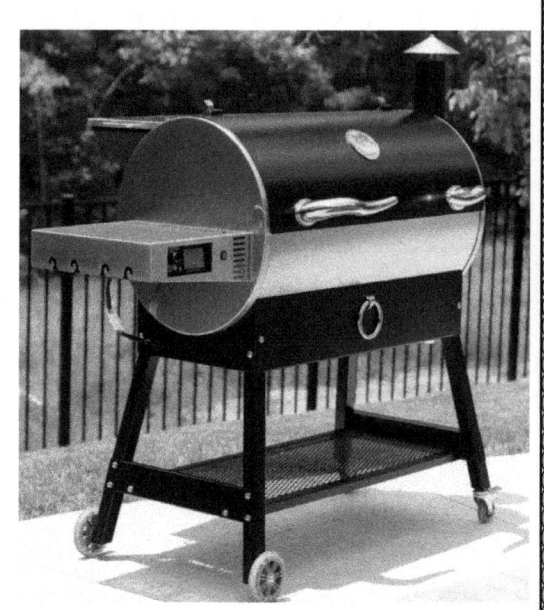

The bulk of the grill is in stainless steel. You also get a large 40 lb. trunk for up to 40 hours of continuous cooking and wheels in the rollerblade style to move the grill around quickly.

8. PIT BOSS 700FB PELLET GRILL — LARGE BUDGET ALTERNATIVE

Pit boss offers a range of pellet grills which is marketed as an inexpensive option to Traeger. You will normally have a couple of hundred fewer grills than your counterpart.

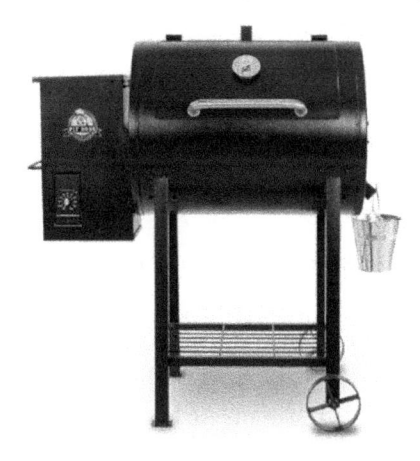

With the 2019 Traegers release, the tech in the Pit Boss is lagging, but the Pit Boss could still be a good buy if you don't care for the latest bells and whistles.

The Pit Boss uses a moving plate device that allows searing easier and more flexible. This grill is remarkably sturdy, given size and weight, with a heavy-handed steel build.

For the SC edition, which comes with an updated cart with a storage case and caster wheels, you can even spend a little extra.

9. WEBER SMOKEFIRE — WEBER'S FIRST ENTRY INTO THE PELLET GRILL MARKET

We had strong expectations for Weber's new pellet barbecue. All the early indicators seemed like they were going to enhance the construction of the grill and address the usual problems with searing. We bought the larger model EX6, which has a grill area of 1008 square inches. You can also choose a smaller EX4 with 672 square inches.

Although we are still checking this grill, our experience was a mixed bag after a few weeks and largely fits what other reviews have told us.

Although all of the food cooked on the SmokeFire smelled amazing and we didn't witness any dangerous fires like others, there have been several issues keeping this barbecue from its maximum capacity.

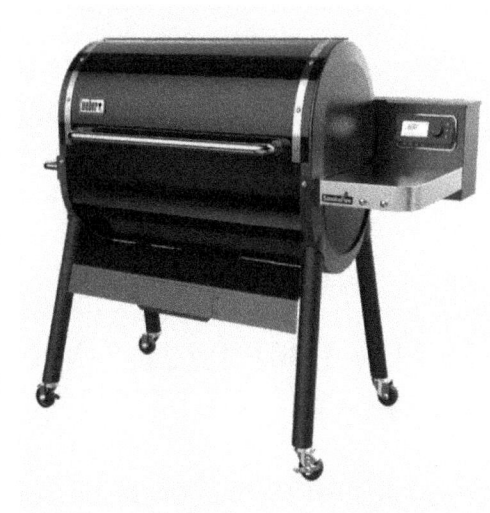

What we liked:

- Searing nice —most pellet grills allow decent smokers and bad grills on average. The Weber SmokeFire architecture helps you to receive a fairly decent sear while cooking at optimum temperature.

- Food has a wonderful taste — while we were rough on this barbecue in our study, every meal we cooked was fantastic too, so at the end of the day, that is the most important aspect.

What we don't like:

- Rushed product introduction — All indicators point towards Weber's early launch and don't invest adequate time monitoring the price.

- Lack of side trays or front cabinet — While it might sound like a Weber, you may purchase an upgrade to repair it; a grill will have some regular room at this price as a default

- Pellet bridge — the hopper configuration appears to protect the pellets from slipping into the furnace, which suggests that they may have to be moved every couple of hours.

- Weak device quality — certain functions were missing when released, but Weber has done a better job in enhancing the iGrill thermometer program, and I think it would still continue to change.

Weber released a free add-on to solve this problem with pellet bridging, so I anticipate that SmokeFire will continue to improve slowly until it becomes one of the best available pellet grills. For decades, Weber has been expanding the gamut of grids since gas and charcoal and it was still hopeful to believe that they will make their first-ever pellet grill attempt.

WHO PELLET SMOKERS ARE BEST SUITED FOR?

Even a pellet smoker at the beginning will give you more back than carbon or gas. But for a bit earlier, you will enjoy the simplicity and versatility that pellet smokers take over the countryside.

It doesn't appear that only two companies made pellet grills long ago. In 2008, you could choose between Traeger and MAK if you wanted to buy a pellet smoker. It's a sign of this type of smoker's popularity that so many new brands can now be chosen.

The prices for decent pellet grills begin at approximately $400 and may surpass $1000. How do you find an outstanding charcoal smoker under 300 dollars like Weber Smokey Mountain? you may ask if you want to purchase a pellet grill.

It takes only two words to sum up the benefits of a pellet smoker's cooking. "Comfort" and "variety."

However, the convenience is fantastic if the price is not a deal-breaker for you. Accustom yourself to throw a wind, fix the temperature, and then run around the day (or sleep the day) with no worries. Since pellet smokers run out of steam, they may also be an excellent alternative whether you stay in a condo or are not lucky enough to be limited to burning charcoal or wood.

HOW PELLET SMOKERS WORK

- Pellet smokers use a very different heat generating system while sharing the 'set and forget' style of their gas and electric cousins.

- Such cigarettes utilize cylindrical wooden cartridges, as the term suggests. A hopper on the side where you place the pellets is a standard setup.

- Once you plug in the grill and adjust the fire to a remote system, the pellets are moved and transformed into fire and smoke. One of the most essential aspects of a pellet smoker is the unit. The machine controls the temperature in your pellet cooker all over the pot.

There are some common kinds of grill controllers:

- Three-position controls: generally found on cheaper pellet cookers, these controls are set to three configurations, low (225°F), medium (325°F) and, high (425°F). We are often referred to as LMH controls. During set intervals, they feed the pellets into the furnace, and you do not have a large amount of temperature power.

- Multi-position controllers: these controls can be used in smaller increments to adjust the temperature. Pellets are fed in set loops that also do not give great precision to these controllers. In optimal settings, a multi-position controller is normally accurate +/-20°F. The inclusion of a Led panel is a good function of these devices.

- Non-PID device with one-touch: This form of control helps you to change the temperature in increments of 5-10°F. In fixed cycles, they still feed pellets, which means that they can only deliver +/-15-20°F accuracy. They also have LCD screens, one-touch buttons, and many have meat sample inputs.

- PID controllers: many found PID controllers to be the gold norm for grill controls. Temperatures are only a few degrees correct. Such method of the device will also handle a programmable meat sample that operates along with the control mechanism to reduce the temperature until the meat is done. The pellet feed is constantly controlled to maintain the right temperature. They do have one-touch buttons and LCD.

DURABILITY AND CONSTRUCTION MATERIAL

Don't be misled by an enticing pellet grill exterior. The maker may have made costs and used inexpensive parts to pick up on the interior, even though there is plenty of stainless steel on the outside.

The most critical components of your grill are the fire bowl, flame deflector, drop bowl, and grates. You have a cooker that lasts a lifetime because such parts are crafted from marine stainless steel.

If you are looking at a BBQ built from stainless steel, make sure it has a really good quality coating. As long as the paint blisters and chips continue to rust, the cooker deteriorates.

It can also be remembered that a pellet smoker made of high-quality materials is safer. High-quality materials preserve heat, allow more effective use of pellets, and help sustain the temperature during cold weather.

SIZE OF THE HOPPER

Your pellet cooker's hopper is the tub that houses the pellets ready to go into the furnace. The scale of your hopper thus ultimately determines the length of your cooks. Therefore, it proves irritating to settle for a hopper that's too low, as your cooks won't be distant.

As a guide, you will find a pellet grill with a 40-pound hopper at the standard smoking temperatures for about 40 hours. In view of the fact that some cooks take about 20 hours; for example, an 18-pound hopper will be problematic.

And remember, your cooker will use even more fuel to raise the smoker and maintain temperature when you live in a colder climate.

You can buy hopper extensions for your grill pellet. Make sure that the hopper extender you are purchasing is compatible with your pellet smoker and the supplier is healthy.

PLAN HOW MUCH COOKING REAL ESTATE YOU NEED

You have to ask yourself a few questions before you know how big your cooker needs to be. How many people am I going to cook for? Do I plan to cook huge cuts or even a whole pig?

Remember, bigger doesn't mean better always. A large pellet cooker can only mean wasted pellets.

An unusual characteristic of pellet smokers is that the cooking region is also dry. As a rule, there should be no variation in temperature between the top rack and the bottom rack during cooking.

Despite this, let us think about the disparity between the primary cooking area and the total cooking region. The central cooking field applies to the field on the central pot. The overall cooking area takes secondary racks into account.

A broad cooker with a primary cooking area of 500 square inches may, therefore, be of less benefit to you than a cooker with a limited cooking area which includes a primary 450 square inch rack and a secondary 125 square inch rack. When you cannot be bothered to do arithmetic, 575 square centimeters of a total area for cooking.

The bottom line is — make an inventory of what you need and don't presume that it's cheaper.

COMMON FEATURES AND CAPABILITIES

- In comparison to the typical charcoal or offset smokers, a whole lot of bells and whistles may be used with pellet grills. Some of the features you should consider include:

- Wi-Fi: companies are beginning to benefit from the fact that pellet smokers have a design computer inside them. By integrating Wi-Fi, the temperature of your grill can be monitored and controlled from almost anywhere as long as there is internet. Companies such as Green Mountain Grills also provide free software that you can access and use for supreme convenience.

- Meat samples: Some pellet cookers have controlled outputs to allow meat samples to be plugged in directly. You can then see readings taken from your meat easily on your cooker's computer.

- Grilling options: Pellet cookers have a downside in the past because of their lack of grilling capabilities. Some manufacturers have made it possible to grill either by removing part of the diffuser plate or by supplying a special grilling area in the cooker.

- Add-ons: Manufacturers often offer a range of supplements. Check for the standard features and what add-ons are at a surcharge. Some add-ons are offered independently from the manufacturer by companies. If your particular cooker has an essential feature but is not a standard feature, make sure it is available as an add-on before you buy the cooker.

LENGTH OF WARRANTY

In pellet smokers, there are some relatively high-tech components. Moving parts are also available, such as the hammer. This means that your cooker may break down and you may not be able to fix it. Make sure you understand exactly how your warranty is extended, what it will cover, what it is void, and where your smoker will need to get in for any reparations.

Warranties vary among manufacturers, so do not be afraid to ask many questions.

PELLET CONSUMPTION

No one loves a pellet dog; a pellet burner that chews needless pellets.

If your pellet cooker is too thin, the cooker's body loses heat. It uses a lot of pellets to keep the temperature.

You will also use many pellets if the metal is too thick. The walls of a thick smoker act as a 'heat sink.' Heat is removed from the stove and stored in the cooker's walls. So, it takes a lot of pellets to reach the desired temperature in the cooking area. Although thick walls are desirable for certain types of cookers, in pellet smokers they are not required.

Research and discover how many pellets the smoker burns per hour. Everything up to one pound an hour is OK at smoking temperatures. Bruce Bjorkman of MAK, for example, claims that his barbecues only use about ½ pound an hour for the smoke.

BEWARE OF GIMMICKS

There is a thin distinction between the practical inventions and gimmicks in the field of pellet smokers. Companies want to stand out above the rest because of increasing competition between manufacturers.

That's not to say all the features are just gimmicks and should be rejected as such. In the end, you have to worry about whether the pellet smoker apps are of particular value to you.

If the feature is something that you'd consider helpful, is it included at the expense of other more important things like pellet use or durability?

However, if you live in a cold climate and it freezes outdoors, being able to control your cook from inside your warm home may be an appealing feature. If that's the case, then Davy Crockett of Green Mountain Grills might be your ally right up there.

CUSTOMER SERVICE

As expected, Awesome Ribs has excellent customer service value advice, particularly for pellet grills.

A dedicated customer service team will likely exist by buying from a more significant, established company. It also means that if you need their help, the company will probably be down the path for around a few years.

A smaller business will provide more intimate and consistent support on the flipside, and your pellet grill concept really would be familiar to the people you approach

You won't figure out if the company fits in when it comes to consumer care until you pose queries and provide straightforward answers.

PRICE

Pellet grills vary considerably in size. Others will save you several hundred dollars and some will cost you thousands of dollars. A word of advice — do not compare a cheap cooker with a good cooker for results.

A cheap cooker will save you early on, but if it continues to rust, after a few short years you do not get a good warranty, and the customer service does not match, you may spend more cash in the long run.

On the other hand, if you bought all of the bells and whistles but didn't use them, you'll have wasted your hard-earned cash when a cooker that costs less would probably have done the trick.

Please check any of the above information before acquiring a currency. See what you can do with your profession and ask certain questions. Then, what you must do is love your fresh cooker!

Given the wide price range, it's important to decide if you want to buy a pellet smoker. Going through a guide is definitely an ideal way of ensuring you have not forgotten anything.

THE PROS AND CONS OF PURCHASING A SMOKER WITH A PELLET

Because of its convenience and versatility, most people choose a pellet-style smoker. Just like a cigarette, you offer:

- Set it down and forget it, just make sure that the hopper is full of pellets and set your desired temperature, and you don't have to worry about that much else.

- Easy temperature regulation — Some pellet smokers require you to dial up to five degrees at temperature and the device is doing an outstanding job of holding the temperature constant.

THERE ARE ALSO A FEW ADVANTAGES UNIQUE TO COOKING WITH A PELLET SMOKER

- Ultra effective fuel — Pellet smokers with a super-powerful convection fan are close to your home oven, but you waste much less on pellet than on oil.

- Less energy washing — any time you barbecue, charcoal smokers will create a little mess. You would need to clear the fireplace now and again with a pellet grill, but it is uncommon (think about per 60 uses).

MEAT SMOKING AND GRILLING WITH FLAVORED SMOKE WOODS

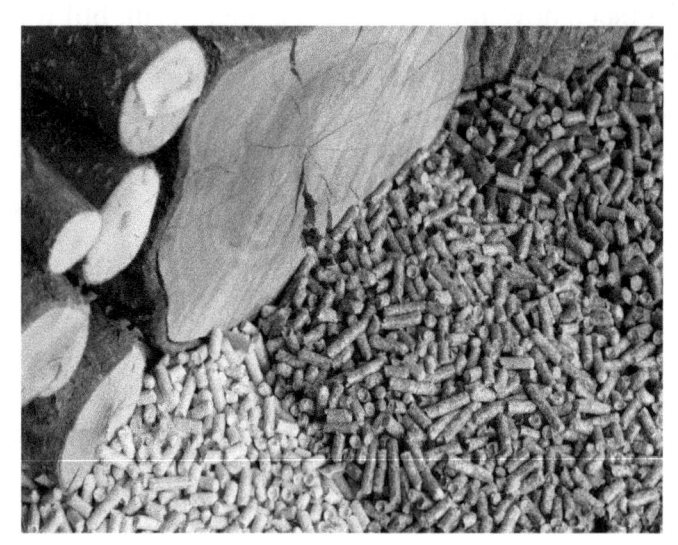

Different Internet reports indicate that all the woods mentioned below are suitable for smoking most beef, poultry, or fish. Oak, hickory, pecan, apple, cherry, and alder are the most popular and widely available fume forests.

Woods to Avoid

Smoking should be cedar, cypress, elm, eucalyptus, black resin, oak, redwood, fir, spruce, citrus, and sycamore. Play it carefully anytime you have a concern regarding a particular smoke wood, before you check from a credible source that it is suitable for use in barbecuing.

Flavored Smoke Woods

Flavored wood chips and chips are sold by retailers. Many were produced from old bottles or barrels of whisky and some were only intoxicated in champagne or sometimes Tabasco. Flavored woods give the smoke coming from your smoker an enticing scent, but you have to know for yourself if they improve your barbecue taste.

Logs, Slabs, Chunks, Chips, And Pellets

In all these forms, you will find smoke wood available. You will most likely find chunks, chips, and pellets in retail stores. Chunks vary in size from small to fist pieces. Chunks burn slowly and release smoke for a long time and are the best-one users' choice.

Chips burn hot and fast and release a rapid burst of smoke. If you use chips, you have to add them several times during the cooking process, while chunks can only be added once at the beginning.

Should Smoke Wood Be Soaked in Water Before Use?

Some people like to soak wooden pieces in water for at least an hour or overnight. This is not necessary, particularly if large chunks are used. Thanks to the sales of Good-One Smokers, the controlled airflow into the smokers enables the chunks to burn slowly throughout the kitchen. Furthermore, water does not penetrate very much seasoned wood anyway.

Should Bark Be Removed?

Any people clearly believe that the bark is stripped from the wood with smoke and giving their barbecue an awful taste. I recognize one person on the other hand who uses bark for barbecue. I'm not disturbing my wood smoke to extract bark. You will do both ways to see how you can make a difference.

Quantity of Smoke Wood to Use

Too much smoke can be added to meat, which leads to a bitter or overpowering aroma. Overall, in the Good-One Smoker Grills, the average of 2-6 fist-shaped blocks of wood performs well for most meats. You should experiment with different amounts of smoke to find out what works best for you, depending on whether you like heavier or lighter smoke.

For the first time, I consider using fresh smoke wood in a limited amount for a lighter smoke taste. Next time, you will still be able to raise the volume of smoke, but there is no way to save meat that has been over-smoked.

Apply Smoke Wood to The Fire

Here are some of the ways in which people add smoke to the fire. Until use, don't bother soaking wood pieces. It is not necessary as long as you use decent pieces, and water will nevertheless not penetrate seasoned wood very much.

1. Place Smoke Wood on Top of Hot Coals

Used most commonly with the Standard Method when firing cookers. Distribute the pieces uniformly over the lit carbon after the meat has been put in the cooker. You will not get hit with smoke when inserting beef, setting up the polder thermometer, etc. If the Minion method is used, make sure that some wood touches the hot coal immediately to produce smoke.

2. Bury Smoke Wood in Unlit Charcoal

Just when the cooker is shot using the Minion Process. Bury wood chunks in the unlit fire, accompanied by a couple of chunks. Distribute the warm coals uniformly over the unlit fuel so that enough wood touches the warm coals to create smoke instantly.

3. Layering Charcoal and Wood Chips

Since I assume the pieces fire faster and more consistently, I'm not in favor of using wood chips. But some people have put a layer of carbon down in the lower part of the chamber, then a wood chip layer, a layer of charcoal, and so on, until the chamber is filled up.

Choosing the Right Smoke Wood

Choosing the correct sort of smoke is an essential option any time you barbecue. Any wood gives its special taste to cattle, swine, poultry, and seafood. It is also valid that other woods are also correlated with other forms of meat and enhance their consistency.

CONCLUSION

For gas or electronic grills nowadays, it is almost difficult to get the true smoke flavor. They definitely meet a specific purpose, but they are not an alternative if you want your food to taste the rich outdoor smoke. The top-class outdoor gas grills are great for fast food cooking. And indeed, just as you would build a gourmet dinner at with an outdoor gas grill. But if you're searching for this perfect outdoor BBQ experience, then you'll need something else to do it.

The smoker has been around for years and is accessible in many shapes and sizes. Many people associate smokers with large ovens which simultaneously cook large quantities of meat. This was and continues to be a growing feature of the giant smoker. To the majority of us who cater to 200 people, we need something more besides a whole side of beef.

The pellet grill is one of the strongest options I have used. What's a barbecue pellet? It looks like your standard outdoor barbecue but is quite different in reality. Next, wood pellets are used for cooking — not gas or charcoal. I also saw other usable pellet fuels like maize. You can use almost any wood you want — hickory, mesquite, cherry, etc. — to get your smoked taste. The other big difference is that the fire is kept away from the food in a firebox. It requires gradual cooking which helps the food to consume the taste of smoke. It's like eating convection.

For certain versions, the pellet fuel will be put into a storage bin and pumped into the barbecue automatically to keep the fire burning. The findings are amazing. You can cook any type of meat, even fish with these grills. I saw cooked biscuits you wouldn't believe. This is a really versatile outside barbecue.

Therefore, you never have to think about gas leakage with these. If you're like me, you've just got a meal halfway through to turn off gas before you're finished. These are also much safer to use than gas, which ensures that they can be washed even better after use.

If you want a unique barbeque experience, look into the pellet grill. When it's time to swap an outdated BBQ or griller, look at a pellet griller before making the next purchase. It will help you to become a true outdoor chef.

Lightning Source UK Ltd.
Milton Keynes UK
UKHW051838180521
383961UK00006B/431